THE NEW
SHIATSU
METHOD

THE NEW SHIATSU METHOD

Helping the Body to Heal Itself

Ryokyu Endo

with Michael Christini & Tzvika Calisar

KODANSHA INTERNATIONAL
Tokyo · New York · London

NOTE FROM THE PUBLISHER: Those with health problems are advised to seek the guidance of a qualified medical or psychological professional before implementing any of the approaches presented in this book. It is essential that any readers who have any reason to suspect serious illness in themselves or their family members seek appropriate medical, nutritional, or psychological advice promptly. Neither this nor any other health-related book should be used as a substitute for qualified care or treatment.

WEBSITE: www.taoshiatsu.com
www.taosangha.com

Calligraphy: Koji Sadamoto.
Model (front cover): Nora Appleton.

Photos by Chiaki Morita, Bunji Adachi, Task Hamazaki, and Haru Sameshima.

Illustrations by Kazuko Ishimaru, Tetsuo Tsukamoto, Masaru Domoto, Jill Segedin, and Megumi Hyuga.

Distributed in the United States by Kodansha America, Inc., and in the United Kingdom and continental Europe by Kodansha Europe Ltd.

Published by Kodansha International Ltd., 17–14 Otowa 1-chome, Bunkyo-ku, Tokyo 112–8652, and Kodansha America, Inc.

No part of this publication may be reproduced in any form or by any means without permission in writing from the publisher.

Copyright © 2004 by Tao Sangha. All rights reserved. Printed in Japan.

First edition, 2004
ISBN 4-7700-2990-X
10 09 08 07 06 05 04   10 9 8 7 6 5 4 3 2 1

www.thejapanpage.com

CONTENTS

FOREWORD by LYALL WATSON   8
INTRODUCTION   10

PART ONE THE KI WORLD — by Ryokyu Endo

1
A NEW APPROACH TO SHIATSU TREATMENT   14

Discovering medical shiatsu   14
Shiatsu in its ideal form   16
Anyone can see ki and meridians   19
The tsubo is a double-edged sword   23
Treating the abnormality—the ideology of Western medicine   24
Seeing the distortion of ki   25
The places where tsubo appear most frequently   26

2
THE TSUBO REVOLUTION IN MERIDIAN MEDICINE   30

How to find tsubo   31
Feeling the echo of the tsubo   33
How to press tsubo   34
The meridians and the ki functions they facilitate   35
Understanding the cause of kyo and jitsu meridians   37
Accessing the kyo meridian   38
Ki is changing each moment   42
Understanding the meaning of tsubo practice   43
Expressing the heart of shiatsu   45

3
THE DEPTHS OF THE KI WORLD 47

EIGHT STAGES TOWARD THE INTERNALIZED DISTORTION OF KI 47

FIRST STAGE Seeing and locating tsubo 47
SECOND STAGE Seeing ki spreading 48
THIRD STAGE Boshin—diagnosing by "looking" 51
FOURTH STAGE Diagnosing the stiffness of the kyo meridian 53

RELEASING THE ENERGY DISTORTION CREATED BY JAKI 54

FIFTH STAGE Discovering the whole-body meridian 54
SIXTH STAGE Seeing the ki body 62
SEVENTH STAGE The existence of the Super Vessels 64
EIGHTH STAGE Jaki and its essence 66

PART TWO ESSENTIAL TAO SHIATSU
— by Michael Christini and Tzvika Calisar

4
THE HEART OF TAO 70

The Five Elements of Tao Shiatsu 70
The heart of sesshin 71
The five-thousand-year-old stream of Oriental medicine 72
Receive Tao ki directly into your heart 73
The power of imagination is the way to receive the Ki Method 74

FIRST ELEMENT **KI DOIN—INCREASE THE POWER AND POTENTIAL OF KI** 75

The principles of Renki 76
FIRST KI PRINCIPLE Synchronization 76
SECOND KI PRINCIPLE Controlling the movement of the tanden 79
THIRD KI PRINCIPLE Using the kidney meridian to strengthen ki 80
FOURTH KI PRINCIPLE Increase speed 81

5
ESSENTIALS OF TREATMENT 82

SECOND ELEMENT PART ONE **THE TSUBO METHOD** 82

The Tsubo Method for effective meridian treatment 82
The way to find ki tsubo 83
The steps in tsubo treatment 84

THIRD ELEMENT **THE KI METHOD FOR SUPER VESSELS AND MERIDIANS**   86

    The Five Aspects of meridian recognition   86
    Locating meridians   89
    Ki Method for the entrance level   90

FOURTH ELEMENT **KYO MERIDIAN TREATMENT**   92

    How to practice kyo meridian treatment   92

6
TREATING INTERNALIZED KI   94

SECOND ELEMENT PART TWO **SUPER VESSEL SPECIFIC TSUBO (SST)**   94

    From folk remedy to medical therapy   94
    Effective medical treatment without sho diagnosis   95
    Ki Method for treatment with the eighteen SST locations   97
    The eighteen SST locations   98

7
WHOLE BODY KI MERIDIAN SHIATSU   106

FIFTH ELEMENT **BASIC FORM**   106

    Basic form supports the kyo deficiency of ki   106
    Ki Method for the Basic Forms   107
    How to develop a program of Five Elements study   116

8
SELF–SHIATSU TREATMENT METHOD   118

    Upper body SST points   119
    Lower body SST points   121

9
KI BREATHING MEDITATION   122

    Responding to the excessive internalization of ki   122
    Healing ki returns to the giver   123
    Ki Breathing meditation   123
    Global ki unification network   125

EPILOGUE   127

FOREWORD

Ryokyu Endo is the internationally renowned master of Tao Shiatsu, which heals the human body at the level of the bioplasm. He is a Buddhist priest of the Pure Land tradition and holds a black belt in the martial art of aikido. In his capacity as a gifted musician, composing and performing on both traditional and modern instruments, he has also created the healing sounds of Tao Music.

The fundamental questions of our existence remain those that ask, "What is 'life'?" and "What is 'death'?" To begin to seek answers to these eternal questions brings us face-to-face with the multiple dimensions that comprise life.

The first is the physiological system with which we are most familiar. Existing in the realm of time and space, it is subject to the physical principles which human investigation has revealed, culminating in the work of Einstein.

The second is that of the spirit or ethereal body. It requires the presence of the physical body for its existence, which is itself dependent, to maintain its health and integrity, on the distribution and regulation of ki. Ki—vital energy—exists at this level, along with the chakra system. Shiatsu and acupuncture's effectiveness is due to their influence at this level.

The energy body belongs to that of the bioplasm at the second level, the bridge between the primary physical level and the third level of the astral body. This is the medium of the soul and spirit at the universal level. We are only just starting to gain a foothold in understanding this level. It is already difficult to find a clear distinction between "life" and "death" here.

Tao Shiatsu and Tao Music affect the level of the bioplasm and reach deeper to the third level, giving us the final state of healing. The melodies of Tao Music surround us with a heavenly peace and the sense of the blossoming of golden flowers from the depths of the Universe. They enable us to discover our true selves at every moment, as we are able to relax by leaving life up to the vast eternal void that is beyond life and death. The melodies are able to create this feeling, as is Tao Shiatsu therapy, because they affect this, the deepest level.

Human beings in the modern age are increasingly wired into a global computer network that surrounds and interconnects the whole earth. Yet ironically, the distortions and stresses of urban living cut people off from the direct experience of the earth as Gaia, as one single living entity.

The healing that Tao Shiatsu and Tao Music bring is for all who suffer and wish to be healed. It is for everyone.

Lyall Watson

INTRODUCTION

Sometimes in life, a moment occurs where you see suddenly the entire world in a different light. Afterwards, things never look quite the same again. This happened to me while giving shiatsu treatment in 1983. The ever-changing pattern of the patient's ki began to reflect as an image. It was as clear as a glass of water sitting on a table. When I responded through the shiatsu to the "stream of ki" I was seeing, the symptom disappeared. It was so dramatic I was shocked.

Oriental medicine studies the flow of ki in the body. Meridians are the channels through which ki moves. Ki is in constant movement, and pain and disease are understood to result from blockages in the movement of ki. When these blockages are released, ki is able to move freely and the symptoms are relieved. Frequently I am asked, "What is ki?" How can something that has no form be explained? It's much like being asked, "What is heart or spirit?" or "What is life?" Ki might be described as vital life energy, created by the underlying unity of heart and body. Since the Meiji period (1868–1912), a time of extensive reform in Japan, much discussion has taken place as to whether ki and meridians really exist. However, as I described, I actually saw the meridian flowing as a line of ki. It was completely different from daily life perception: the eye to behold another dimension had opened. Since that day I began to enter into the infinite world of ki.

Many people in the West wonder if ki and meridians really exist. Ki seems so far removed from "real" life that they feel it must be something supernatural or open to just a handful of people with special abilities. Even in Japan there has been debate about the existence of ki. In fact, ki is everywhere and accessible to every one of us. But like the air we breathe, it's too close for all of us to even notice. It wasn't until after my heart opened that I could see ki. Then I began to experience a world completely different from what I had previously known in daily life. I began to explore the infinite world of ki.

According to the Gaia hypothesis, earth and life (all life, not only human life) form a single, connected, self-regulating unit. The connector is what we call ki in Japanese. The constant, universal movement of ki affects and unites all organic existence. In other words, at the deepest level of existence, heart, mind, body, and matter are one. This is a core principle in Oriental philosophy and medicine, and now quantum theory and advances in scientific measurement are beginning to confirm it.

We have entered an age where the focus of human consciousness has shifted, and is moving away from materialism toward spirituality. The turning point was in 1985.

I experienced the change, quite literally, through my skin, while practicing and teaching shiatsu all over the world. The hearts of students I was teaching began to open, allowing them to recognize tsubo (meridian treatment points) empathetically. In Japan, Israel, the United States, New Zealand, Australia, and Europe, students began to respond to the world of ki and meridians.

Ki and meridians belong to the world of the subconscious, and it was at this level that the initial shift took place. Changes in the heart state and consciousness of people followed.

By the new millennium, hearts and consciousness had opened even further, reducing our dependence on material existence as the primary basis for human relations.

In the future, society's direction in economics, industry, and culture will also shift. Looking at the environment leads us to realize that many current practices must change. A similar shift will improve health care and medical treatment. The focus of medicine will move toward holistic meridian medicine, based on the unfolding of the heart.

Modern Western medicine, with its reliance on surgery, strong drugs, and advanced technology, can be dramatically effective. Emerging technologies, like genomics and proteomics, offer the possibility of effective treatment for major diseases in narrowly specific circumstances.

But high-tech medicine has failed to solve the greatest problem confronting it: the growing late twentieth-century plague of chronic, debilitating diseases. These diseases are not immediately life threatening, but they destroy quality of life and cause great suffering. I believe Tao Shiatsu, the medicine of ki, is responding and adapting to these changes in illness. The dawn of its spiritual culture can already be glimpsed. I believe the sunrise of the human heart is on the horizon.

This book is an attempt to explain what the ki world is like, how it works and what kind of heart makes it possible to see ki and enter into this world. Much has been written about ki, but usually from an occult angle, or based on analyses of ancient Oriental medical classics. This book is the story of my personal and clinical experience with ki over the last quarter century.

Ryokyu Endo

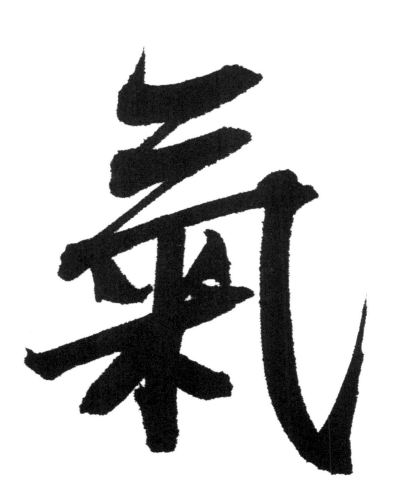

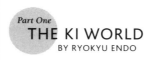

Part One
THE KI WORLD
BY RYOKYU ENDO

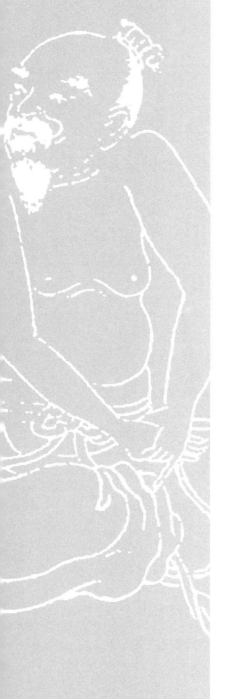

1

A NEW APPROACH TO SHIATSU TREATMENT

DISCOVERING MEDICAL SHIATSU

A holistic understanding of the interconnected nature of all life underlies the philosophy of Taoism and Tao Shiatsu. Just as a drop of rain becomes a stream, then flows into a river and finally fills an ocean, a new way of approaching tsubo and shiatsu treatment began with just one idea. This, then, is the story of the journey from that one idea.

The purpose of my initial study of shiatsu in 1976 at the Japan Shiatsu School was to pass the national examination, in order to get a license to practice. Many graduates of this test shared my doubts as to whether the qualification had any value. Our training consisted of nothing more than learning how to give treatment for relaxation to make people feel good. Even today, this is still a common perception many people have of shiatsu's purpose. The techniques we were taught focused on the physical body alone. Tsubo, or treatment points, were seen merely as places to apply pressure. If enough points were pressed, some might hit the right spot. This approach was applied for all symptoms.

My first experience with shiatsu had occurred while I was playing guitar in a rhythm and blues band. I had dropped out of high school for the second time, much like the character Holden in *Catcher in the Rye*, and was playing with a band in Tokyo nightclubs. The bassist occasionally gave me shiatsu that he had learned from a book. I was amazed how much comfort it gave me. This experience had the same kind of impact on me as forming my first band in high school, and starting intensive aikido practice. The book the bassist was referring to was *Do It Yourself—Three Minute Shiatsu*, by Tokujiro Namikoshi. In it the author describes how he successfully treated Marilyn Monroe for a stomach disorder during her visit to Tokyo, cured his mother's arthritic pain, and founded the Japan Shiatsu School, where I was to study first. Reading Namikoshi's book left me wondering if a world such as this really existed. My excitement led me on a search for similar books, but I soon discovered that not many existed at the time. I studied those that I could lay my hands on and they inspired my first efforts to give shiatsu to people and enroll in his school. However, my life didn't change significantly after graduating and receiving a license to practice.

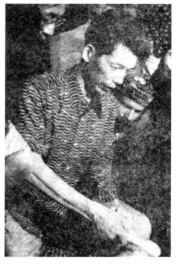

Master Masunaga and the author (upper left).

A major change occurred when I attended the Zen Shiatsu school of Master Shizuto Masunaga in 1980. The Iokai Center in Tokyo was where Master Masunaga taught the Zen Shiatsu therapy he had founded. In returning to the origins of Oriental medicine, he had re-established the first systematic form of diagnosis for shiatsu. This involved determining accurately which meridians to treat in order to provide the most effective relief of the patient's symptoms. He performed this by palpating the meridian diagnosis points that he had identified and mapped in the *hara* (abdominal region), through his ability to visualize the meridian stream. Master Masunaga had also created a way of treating that was very different from the orthodox technique I had learned. Instead of relying solely on the thumbs and fingers, the forearms and knees were also utilized, with movement of the practitioner's whole body directing pressure. Its inherently holistic approach used supporting pressure, coupled with the leaning of the practitioner's body weight toward the patient to apply therapeutic pressure.

Zen Shiatsu was remarkably different from the techniques that relied on applying pressure with muscular strength. Additionally, Master Masunaga's philosophical understanding and theoretical teaching about meridians astounded us. The seminars, classes, and clinical demonstrations of the medical effectiveness of his treatment left me greatly impressed. The depth of Oriental medicine was revealed. Sadly, as it turned out, it was not long before Master Masunaga's death. During the time I spent studying with him, I never imagined that these would be his last classes. All those who witnessed his teaching were deeply moved. Zen Shiatsu's growth around the world is the legacy of what he accomplished.

Experiencing this and witnessing the effectiveness of the treatment motivated me to begin researching the meridians. I was filled with an almost childlike curiosity and newfound focus and concentration. There was a feeling of having "dropped into" this journey of researching medical shiatsu, the core of Oriental medicine. In light of this experience, my previous shiatsu studies for the national certificate seemed, more than ever, mere techniques for relaxation and pleasure. What I now embarked upon was continuous clinical research for increasing the effectiveness of treatment. Developing this method of medical shiatsu was a boundless journey without a fixed goal. However, after a while, I found that the road had come to a dead end.

SHIATSU IN ITS IDEAL FORM

The reason for this was the inability to perform accurate diagnosis. By diagnosis I do not mean the Western medical approach of categorizing and naming the patients' symptoms or disease. Diagnosis in the Oriental sense involves determining which of the energy meridians requires treatment in order to stimulate the body's internal healing response, and so return the energetic system to a state of equilibrium.

Shortly after commencing Master Masunaga's classes, I began to practice what I was learning. This involved first giving a basic shiatsu sequence to the whole body. This was then followed by treatment to the flow of energy, or ki stream, in the meridian that seemed to be energy deficient in relation to the other meridians: this is called the *kyo* meridian. However, I was not able to be certain that the meridian selected—the diagnosis—was in fact accurate. From what I have observed while teaching around the world, this is the case for most people who practice Zen Shiatsu. From the point where the road stopped in my research, three years were to pass before I became able to see or visualize the kyo meridian, but this development enabled me to relieve the symptoms of significantly more patients. I will discuss this mechanism in greater detail in chapter three.

Shiatsu is a truly wonderful gift for humanity and a core manual therapy of Oriental medicine. The ki stream is the real essence of this core. What makes it possible to visualize this stream of ki as Master Masunaga did? I have reflected a great deal on this while researching and teaching shiatsu in Japan and around the world. Zen Shiatsu is not particularly well known in Japan—a fact that surprises many Western practitioners, most of whom use Master Masunaga's style of shiatsu. Previously in the West, the classical or Namikoshi style of shiatsu (that I studied initially) had been the most widespread, as it still is in Japan today. However, this gradually changed as the many Western students who had studied at Masunaga's Iokai Center returned to their countries.

What then is the current situation of Zen Shiatsu in the West? One impression I have gathered from Western students attending my seminars and workshops is that shiatsu schools and federations in the West readily accept (and sometimes teach) that if there are ten practitioners, ten different diagnoses may result. Is this genuinely acceptable, or merely an excuse? If this situation is widely accepted, then it would appear that the only significant change to the basis of shiatsu practice is using the forearms and knees in addition to the techniques of the hands and thumbs. This is far removed from the ideal of Zen Shiatsu. Is there an alternative to this situation?

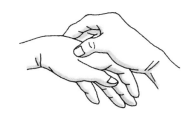

Pressing tsubo as a fixed point.

In Japan the word *tsubo*, or treatment point, is well known, but anyone with real knowledge of this word is likely to be a specialist and would use the equivalent acupuncture term *keiketsu*. While many books have been written about these treatment points, they tend to approach the subject from the perspective that if you press a certain point in a fixed location, it will have an effect on a corresponding condition. For example, a book will show a point located on the hand in the area between the thumb and index finger, and will state that pressing that point will relieve constipation. Even people who are not practitioners are familiar with this kind of information.

This concept of tsubo is derived from acupuncture. It is prescriptive; treatment for specific symptoms is associated with specific points. I have always had mixed feelings about this approach, half believing and half doubting. When giving treatment this way, I frequently found that pressing a tsubo that was located as a fixed point produced no response and gave no benefit to the patient.

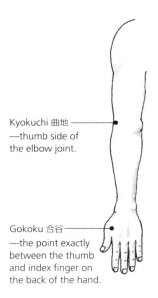

Kyokuchi 曲地 —thumb side of the elbow joint.

Gokoku 合谷 —the point exactly between the thumb and index finger on the back of the hand.

Tsubo as named and numbered fixed points.

One day I ignored this approach and instead imagined where the patient most wanted to be pressed. This led me to find a physical depression that had at its center something that felt like the tip of a rice grain. This is how it felt. To understand more clearly what the nature of this was, I questioned the patient while pressing the "rice tip." A common response was that this was the point they really wanted to be pressed. While continuing to press, I imagined how the patient was feeling and adapted the pressure moment to moment. I did this according to the receiver's response until the rice tip disappeared. Most people receiving this treatment commented how comfortable it was. Sometimes the rice tip "echoed." This sensation was like an electric current traveling to the symptom or place where pain was felt. After the echo became less or finished traveling to the symptom's location, the pain disappeared. This seemed to me to be the real meaning of tsubo.

I researched this new way of giving shiatsu through the treatments I was giving, and I saw a dramatic improvement in my patients' symptoms. So there seemed to be real value in working this way. Both practitioner and patient could really feel something. Some of these tsubo locations were similar to keiketsu (acupuncture treatment points), but many were different.

The location and the strength of the effect and echo in the patient's body (the tsubo's depth) also differed from person to person, and from treatment to treatment.

This is exactly how it should be if tsubo are in fact an expression of the individual's life force. Life itself is unceasing change: tsubo are a manifestation of this. Tsubo reveal the constantly changing life stream. Empathetic imagination must always guide any connection to tsubo, and practitioners must constantly strive to develop the capacity to imagine how their patient is subconsciously feeling. This involves checking if the response to pressure is comfortable or not, asking if there is any echo, and continually confirming these points while treating.

In his book *The Method of Health with Meridian and Tsubo,* Master Masunaga wrote, "Tsubo is more than point, more than location." Perhaps in this sentence we can see his understanding of the real nature of tsubo. There was almost nothing else that I could find written that reflected this approach to tsubo. What I had discovered, almost by coincidence as the result of going with a single idea, was that tsubo are not in fixed locations. I had wanted to see where this would lead. Continuing to follow this way of treating resulted in a significant increase in treatment effectiveness. For the practitioner who cannot accurately diagnose the meridians, I feel this is the only way to give medically effective shiatsu treatment.

So three years passed and my research continued in this manner: locating and treating the rice tip by empathetic imagination. Simply stated, this involved imagining where the receiver most wanted to be pressed and, while pressing, imagining each moment how the receiver was feeling. It was while working in this way that I went one summer to assist at the clinic of a former classmate from Masunaga's Iokai Center. This was when the big shift in my consciousness occurred. It happened suddenly without warning as I was treating a patient's tsubo located in the hara (abdomen), where an internal organ problem existed. As I glanced at the hara I "saw" the kyo meridian, the meridian that most needed to receive ki. To begin with it was hazy, but little by little it became clear. Based on this image, I gave treatment to the kyo meridian through its channel in the arms and legs. The patient reported that the pain and symptom had disappeared.

This was the same phenomenon of instant effectiveness that we had witnessed with Master Masunaga's treatment. In that moment, the truth of Master Masunaga's teachings on meridian medicine was completely confirmed. At the time of studying with him, I hadn't been able to rid myself of an element of doubt about the existence of the meridians. Even the person who invited Master Masunaga to teach in the United States had asked me: "Is it really true what Master Masunaga says about meridians, do they actually exist?"

Branches of acupuncture, and even some shiatsu schools, have said that the meridians and tsubo are just a superstition of the ancient Chinese. Much of the acupuncture practiced in Japan is based on scientific rationale and disregards the existence of the meridians in its practice. I cannot laugh at or criticize this because I, too, once wondered whether the meridians really existed. Human beings have a tendency to think only about the things that they can understand, and it is easy for people to dismiss things that are difficult to understand. Meridians do exist. It was just not until something deep inside me shifted and opened the window to my heart* that I could see them.

> * *Kokoro* and *shin* 心
>
> *Kokoro* and *shin* are Japanese terms that can only be encompassed in English, depending on the context, by a combination of the words heart, mind, spirit, feeling, and emotion. The word "heart" does not completely capture the essence of *kokoro* or *shin*, so when used here, it expresses the concept of heart–mind with the aspect of spirit. This is the supporting foundation of the physical body, and is projected through it by intention of thought and feeling in the form of ki.

By simply following the kyo meridian diagnosis—that is, giving shiatsu to the meridian most deficient in ki—an amazing increase in the effectiveness of treatment resulted. In addition, treatment became much more relaxing when free from the tension created by the uncertainty about which meridian to treat. Then, inexplicably, every night for one week following this revelation, words and sentences from Master Masunaga's lectures echoed repetitively in my mind. It was just like a tape or video recorder playing. When I had listened to these words in the lectures, I had only been able to understand them intellectually. After what had just happened, though, I could now understand the full depth of the words and their real meaning. Every night I was saying to myself, "Oh, that's what he meant." I realized the vast gap that had existed between what my head had understood and this real understanding.

ANYONE CAN SEE KI AND MERIDIANS

When I glanced at the patient's hara, as described earlier, the distortion of the patient's ki appeared as clearly as a glass of water sitting on a table. It left me thinking, could this really be true? But the results could not be argued with. It was clear: look at the meridian—the source of life—and read its ki, then pain and symptoms can be easily and completely cured with shiatsu treatment. If the patient's ki responds to the practitioner's, then this is what happens. I was truly surprised at the effectiveness.

What I was doing felt in some ways very mysterious: experiencing the real *sho* diagnosis of the meridians. Sho diagnosis is fundamental to all branches of Oriental medicine and determines the excess (*jissho*) and deficiency (*kyosho*) of ki energy in the meridians. This allows the practitioner to determine what stimulation of the meridian's ki stream is required to return the patient's life to a holistic state of wellness. The next realization was that this was not a manifestation of supernatural power. The mechanism of Oriental healing described by Master Masunaga occurs when the patient's ki responds to the giver's ki. When it occurs without knowledge of the mechanism, it must seem like a miracle. Over many years my heart had been moving toward a deep subconscious shift in understanding. The ki world is directly connected to the subconscious realm of existence, rather than the relatively more superficial level of consciousness. Time is required for any shift in subconscious perception to come up to the surface level of consciousness.

Over the past twenty-five years of research, I have spent a lot of time teaching people of different cultures both in Japan and abroad. It takes much more time, effort, and energy to be aware of what I'm doing subconsciously in order to explain it to people in another language. In Japan there is a saying, "There is no second generation in a great master's time." This is not because the master does not wish to teach all he knows, but rather that the life of the master will usually end before he is able to teach the method effectively. To be able to explain to others what it is that you are doing is not an easy task. In some ways I was lucky to have been teaching outside of my own country and having to use a different language,

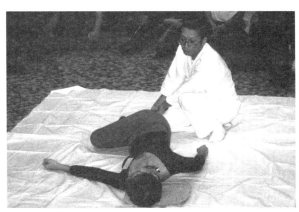 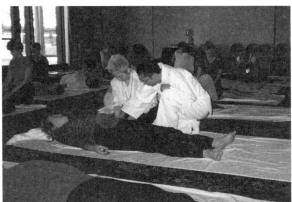

The author demonstrating Tao Shiatsu clinical treatment at an International Shiatsu conference in Berlin (left), and showing the correct location of the Bladder meridian to Pauline Sasaki at the Tao Shiatsu workshop in the AOBTA convention (right).

since this enabled me to systematize the teaching in words much more quickly in order to overcome any language barrier.

During this period of research and building up the teaching system, a real shift took place in what I call the "time age." The expression of human ki through the meridian system has changed dramatically since the mid-1980s, as I will fully explain in chapter three. This proved to be an opportunity to re-evaluate the practice of manual therapy, which led to a marked increase in treatment effectiveness through the methods of Tao Shiatsu. Now this turning point in human history has been reached, the world will experience major physical shifts in many forms. Take, for example, the greatest means of transportation of our time. People in the future will look back upon the fossil fuel-powered car with horror. From their solar or hydrogen-powered vehicles they will ask, "What kind of people would have used a means of transport whose fuel polluted the very air they breathed—how could they have done that? How primitive they were!" However, before the physical world changes, the ki world will change first. The ki distortion in human beings increased dramatically before the turning point was reached. I was able to feel and experience this around the world while teaching in many different countries. Tao Shiatsu offers a previously unknown treatment and teaching system that is capable of healing the distortions in the human meridian system, created by the changes of this age.

My attempt to find treatment solutions to the challenges presented by the changes in the meridian system was greatly assisted, as I said earlier, by teaching in different countries and cultures. It created a synchronization that took me deeper and deeper into the ki world. One example is the discovery of the Super Vessels that are utilized in Tao Shiatsu treatment, of which there is no mention in the classics. They will be explained in detail in chapter three, but essentially they are meridians that exist at a depth of seven meters beyond the physical body. This is, of course, completely beyond commonsense understanding. Yet it is due to this depth that they can be felt on the surface of the body, having an almost physical existence that can be touched and felt by anyone. The phenomena of the ki world, in truth, are no less a part of reality than the things perceived in daily life at the commonsense level. When my heart opened enabling me to see ki, I was given the opportunity to experience the phenomena that exist beyond common sense. I continually had to ask myself whether this was just my own personal understanding or not, and seek confirmation. The responsibility I feel toward teaching shiatsu means I could never knowingly teach something that I wasn't sure was right. I have always therefore confirmed the effectiveness of a method first through my clinical practice, and then with other Tao Shiatsu practitioners.

At the point when I realized that the Super Vessels could be recognized simultaneously on the body's surface with daily life consciousness, and at the deepest level of the ki or energetic body surrounding the physical form, I also recognized the depth of what I call the "heart world." This is the basis of each individual's life, just as the Tao, the Spirit of the Universe, is the source and base of all existence. It is the heart state that is creating, projecting, and shifting our conscious existence. The system of Tao Shiatsu became clear with this realization. Everything seemed to be synchronized as people began to understand more deeply the world of ki existing beyond our common perception. It brought to mind the idea of the collective unconscious in Jungian psychology. Oriental medical philosophy teaches that the body is holistically one. The inner heart and external world are like a mirror to one another, constantly reflecting each other. The revelations of the ki world, such as the Super Vessels, allowed me to actually see and feel this reality. It also opened my eyes to the illusionary nature of common sense and the awareness that reality is not limited to what is recognized by natural science. The ki world cannot be comprehended through the rationale of natural science, yet my research shows that it consists of eight different depths, which are explained in detail in chapter three.

Human consciousness is undergoing a dramatic shift. All levels and aspects of life, including medicine, are affected since all life exists as an interconnected whole. The commonsense approach to Oriental medicine derived from the classics has outlived its usefulness. Especially in regards to tsubo, my respect and trust in how they are commonly understood declined to the point where I had to accept that they no longer had any meaning for clinical shiatsu practice.

In shiatsu classes, I began to teach this new form of tsubo therapy. My expectation was that people would be able to give effective treatment with it, so I was amazed and then somewhat disappointed when hardly anyone understood what I was talking about. Only a few people could feel the tsubo, or rice tip, and I soon realized why. They were trying to feel the sensation of the rice tip by using their physical sense of touch to reveal the presence of tsubo, and this is not possible: only with the primal sense can it be experienced. In Japanese, the kanji for "touch" is *shoku* (触). It is made up of different elements, one of which signifies an insect's antenna, the sensor used to judge if the outside is dangerous or not. Basically, our skin performs the same function in conjunction with the brain via the sense of touch. This discriminating sense allows us to recognize objects that exist outside of us. By comparison, the sensation of the rice tip is experienced with a different part of the brain. It is an empathizing sense that allows us to identify with someone in pain and prompts us to help them. The sense of touch and the primal sense have a seesaw type of relationship, much

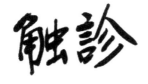

The kanji for *shokushin*.

like the sympathetic and parasympathetic (autonomic) nervous systems: when one becomes stronger the other becomes weaker. The discriminating sense of touch often becomes stronger when someone is highly developed at the calculations required in daily living. Consequently, the empathizing primal sense is diminished, which can leave them unable to identify with and feel another person's suffering. Likewise, when the naturalness and simplicity of the primal sense is rich, a person is more likely to be open and responsive to the feelings and life sensation of others.

THE TSUBO IS A DOUBLE-EDGED SWORD

For treatment to be effective, the tsubo must be felt with empathetic imagination. If people attempt to touch and press tsubo as physical matter, then harm to the patient's ki may result. Even though I teach this over and over, many students in class still persist with the physical approach. I've tried

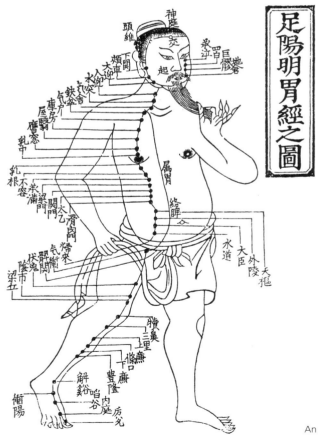

An ancient meridian diagram.

many ways to teach tsubo so that everybody understands, and for a while I even gave up and stopped teaching tsubo. I believe that Master Masunaga never talked about tsubo in class because he realized that people would not understand the real depth of the teaching. Over time, though, something very interesting started to happen. Ordinary people began talking about ki and meridians, and these ideas began to be accepted. Recently all kinds of people are talking about ki, not just specialists in this field. In seminars around the world, people are now able to feel the rice tip from the very first day.

Much of the approach of modern-day Oriental medicine has fallen into the trap presented by the commonsense view of natural science. I've wanted for some time to talk about this and how it is related to the previous discussion of tsubo. The acupuncture points of three thousand years' standing, represented in the well-known charts by names and numbers, are one of the falsehoods of Oriental medicine. This is a strong statement to make, so please allow me to explain further. In this system, each tsubo is assigned to the treatment of a particular disease or condition. However, the real nature of diagnosis and treatment in Oriental medicine is not necessarily to put a name to the disease or condition: seeking to do so is a requirement of Western medical diagnosis. Categorizing differences in symptoms, however, is not an absolute or universal approach. Oriental medicine takes a completely different point of view. In order to understand this difference more clearly, it is helpful to look at the ideas and concepts that are the foundations of Western medicine.

TREATING THE ABNORMALITY —THE IDEOLOGY OF WESTERN MEDICINE

The professed intention of Oriental medicine is to understand the imbalance in ki by determining in which meridians there is a relative excess and deficiency in ki: this is known as the *sho diagnosis*. By following this, the practitioner is able to provide the appropriate stimulation of the patient's ki to help it return to a holistic state, which is described as "returning to nature." Western medicine in its approach seeks to treat the part that is deemed to be sick or abnormal, thus the aim of diagnosis is to find the place or part where something is wrong. Treatment options then focus on either surgery to remove or correct the diseased or malfunctioning part, or drug therapy to support any chemical deficiency or excess by administering usually synthetic chemical compounds.

Western medical concepts, I believe, have literally brainwashed us to such an extent that when we hear the word medicine, or medical treatment, we automatically think of treatment as being applied to the part or place that is deemed to be bad. Oriental medicine looks at the body from a different perspective, not simply as "matter," with separation of mind and body. Due to this entirely different point of view, disease is also viewed very differently. Oriental medicine does not look for the bad part as the cause of disease. It approaches diagnosis through understanding the state of the patient's ki—the holistic oneness that exists in every part of the body.

Asking the question, "Where is the abnormality?" has no purpose in Oriental medical diagnosis. Rather, questions are posed such as, "With what stimulation can the patient's life force be expected to respond and heal itself?" and "By what means will the self-healing ki of the patient be awoken?" This means the diagnosis consists of asking the questions to guide the therapy itself. Diagnosis is itself part of the treatment. The doctor in Western medicine is making the diagnosis as an observer looking at the body as a physical phenomenon, from a supposedly objective point of view. This mirrors the requirements that form the methodology of scientific experimentation. Oriental medicine cannot stand in that position.

SEEING THE DISTORTION OF KI

Accepting and then experiencing that ki can only be seen through the unification of the object and subject is a prerequisite to understanding Oriental medical diagnosis. It can only occur in a relationship of oneness between the practitioner and patient. In Tao Shiatsu this is called *ki unification*. Even now, experiments in the field of quantum physics are revealing that it is impossible to separate the observer from what is being observed. This finding is at odds with the objective observation of phenomena that has been the basis of scientific experimentation and research. These discoveries have the potential to erode one of the pillars that supports natural science and has strong implications for Western medicine.

Diagnosis is in itself part of the treatment in Oriental medicine. By contrast, in Western medicine, diagnosis must take place before treatment can commence. A doctor faced with a patient in a Western clinical setting in which there is no identifiable problem or abnormality, is often rendered powerless to provide treatment. The doctor is faced with the problem of what action to take. Sometimes, even with a diagnosis, there may be no treatment option available. This is almost never the case in Oriental medicine.

In herbal therapy, for example, diagnosis reveals the name of the herb that will bring about the self-healing response in the patient. Understanding the patient's ki empathetically is the means by which the most accurate herbal combination and dosage for the particular individual is prescribed. Diagnosis in shiatsu treatment may reveal the Large Intestine meridian to be kyo, but this does not mean that there is something wrong with this meridian. From the diagnosis we can expect that giving shiatsu to this meridian will provide the stimulation to return heart, mind, and body to a state of wholeness. Diagnosis includes what strength of shiatsu should be applied, the degree and timing of pressure, and the adaptation of the treatment to the constantly changing ki stream of the meridian.

According to Oriental medicine, disease or illness is a reflection of the disturbance in ki and the associated distortion of the meridians. Finding those tsubo that are able to release this distortion and so relieve the patient's suffering is the real essence of shiatsu and acupuncture. Without seeing the distortion in ki and responding to it as the focus of treatment, the situation arises where points are needled or pressed according to a symptomatic assessment. Treatment then proceeds in a formulaic, almost mathematical manner. Again, this cannot be called Oriental medicine.

THE PLACES WHERE TSUBO APPEAR MOST FREQUENTLY

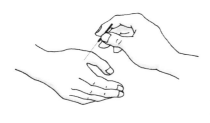

Acupuncture needle insertion.

Tsubo do not exist as points with a fixed location. This may be at odds with what is expressed in the classical texts and with the way acupuncture is practiced today. However, if tsubo are approached as fixed points, shiatsu in particular cannot conform to the philosophy and spirit of Oriental medicine. Even acupuncturists I know performing shiatsu are willing to admit that treating tsubo in the same way as acupuncture points is severely limiting and mistaken in shiatsu treatment.

Tsubo were recorded as fixed points in the classics and this came to be accepted as doctrine. Let us look at the reasons for this. In the classics much discussion takes place about "prohibited points," along with cautions about inserting needles into them. They state that doing so would result in the person's death within a period of so many days, depending on the point and the duration of insertion. If a doctor performing acupuncture was not adequately experienced or trained, then a real risk existed from the mistaken insertion of a needle. To prevent this from happening, the locations of tsubo were fixed. It was obviously necessary that these points were therapeutically effective, thus the locations chosen were those where the probability of tsubo appearing was the greatest. These locations were no doubt influenced by the prevailing medical conditions of the age.

The distortion in ki manifests itself differently in each historical period. In my own clinical experience, for example, from 1989 up to fifty percent of all diagnoses revealed the kyo meridian to be the Conception Vessel.

THE TAO SHIATSU TWENTY-FOUR MERIDIANS CHART

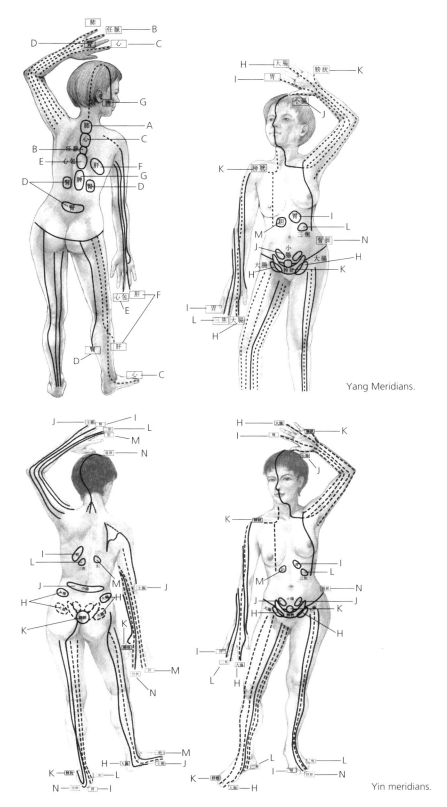

Yang Meridians.

Yin meridians.

A. Lung
B. Conception Vessel
C. Heart
D. Kidney
E. Heart Constrictor
F. Liver
G. Spleen
H. Large Intestine
I. Stomach
J. Small Intestine
K. Bladder
L. Triple Heater
M. Gallbladder
N. Governer Vessel

A NEW APPROACH TO SHIATSU TREATMENT

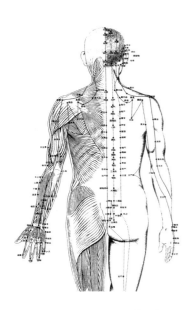

The acupuncture tsubo chart.

The Conception Vessel and Governor Vessel are extra channels and additional to the twelve major meridian channels used in treatment. I found this to be the case no matter where in the world I was giving treatment. Both in Japan and in the many countries I have taught and given treatment in, clinical observation linked this marked increase in Conception Vessel kyo to the meridian system's response to a general weakening of the human immune system. Around the autumn of 1999, the marked pattern of Conception Vessel kyo began to shift to a predominance of Large Intestine and Governor Vessel kyo. It is thus my belief that locations of tsubo in the classics were fixed at a time when the greatest possibility existed that tsubo would appear in those locations. In China, many new tsubo other than those in the classics are now being used. This reflects the changing conditions of the age, and the associated condition of the meridians.

This leads us on to a discussion of the meridian chart. What I have had the privilege to experience with meridians leads me to believe that the classical meridian chart is inaccurate and contains many errors. The classical view is of twelve meridians, six flowing in the arms and six in the legs. In fact there are twenty-four meridians (twelve meridians plus their twelve sub meridians), each of which flows both in the arms and legs. Furthermore, the charts used in acupuncture show meridians that switch direction at unnaturally sharp angles, often back and forth. No meridians flow like that, however. As my clinical experience has confirmed, and as you would expect from observing the flow of other natural phenomena, the meridian stream flows with very natural curves.

So many aspects of the meridian network necessary for deeply effective meridian treatment today are missing from the classics. Only one ring or horizontally flowing meridian is shown, an extra meridian called *taimyaku* in Japanese. In fact, each meridian stream has numerous ring lines and two spiral lines that are not described or depicted in the classics. In the classics the Conception and Governor Vessels are each shown to have only a center line, with Conception flowing on the front of the torso, while Governor flows on the back. In Tao Shiatsu both these meridians have streams in the arms and legs, and are fully utilized in clinical practice.

The classical meridians alone are no longer sufficient for the current age, and the incorporation of this new knowledge of the meridians is absolutely necessary to fulfill the treatment needs of patients. This is no different from how it would have been at the time the classics were written. At that time, it was the full expression of the knowledge available to satisfactorily treat the condition of the meridians as they were known then. The meridian chart itself is not depicted in the classics; only the location of the points is described. Acupuncture meridian charts of the type used nowadays show lines that were simply drawn to connect one point to

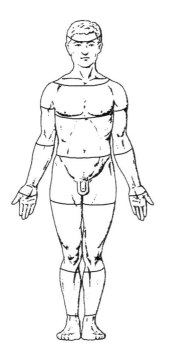
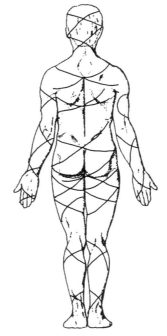

Ring and spiral meridians.

the next. This explains some of the unusual angles. It is also possible that at the time the classics were written, people had already lost the capacity to actually visualize the meridians through the heart state of the primal sense. That is why the tsubo points were depicted as they are.

In addition, in ancient China real knowledge was only transferred by word of mouth and not through books. The secret nature of important knowledge was common. It is written in the classics: "You cannot teach the 'treasures of heaven' (the methods of Oriental medicine) to just anyone." From this we could infer that what was actually written down merely represented the more superficial aspects. This has long been my instinctive feeling while reading the classical texts.

Of course I am curious about how people practicing acupuncture feel about these views. Kohei Kurahara is a Japanese friend who teaches acupuncture at Boston University and who also teaches occasionally at the Boston Shiatsu School where I have given seminars. According to him, acupuncturists who are really trying to give meridian treatment gradually come to understand that the tsubo and meridians do not exist as fixed locations. Currently there is no accepted principle in dealing with how to approach the tsubo in this new way. What seems to hold back deeper understanding is twofold: the presupposition that the classics are absolutely correct and unchanging, coupled with the energy expended in trying to interpret them.

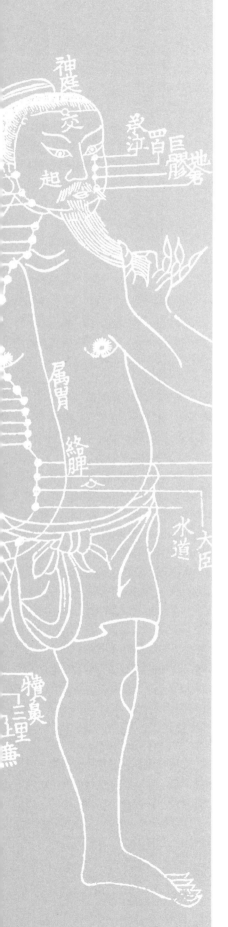

2

THE TSUBO REVOLUTION IN MERIDIAN MEDICINE

The time has come, then, to move beyond the previous concepts of tsubo, and leave behind any doubts about whether they exist or about the effectiveness of tsubo treatment. It never occurred to me that I might one day write about the tsubo of Oriental medicine in the way I am here. My first book—*Tao Shiatsu: Life Medicine for the 21st Century*—began to approach this subject, but not with sufficient confidence that it could be understood, and I therefore found myself writing on a more subconscious level. Humanity is now entering a new era and with it the world of Oriental medicine. The focus can now be on how anyone can locate and treat tsubo. By this I mean that anyone can experience, whether from the position of giver or receiver of tsubo treatment, real medical effectiveness that is in accordance with the principles of Oriental medicine. What is required to do this is an open mind, the motivation to develop the heart that wishes deeply to help others, and the trust to follow the steps exactly as they are set out. There is no need to be a medical professional to do this.

Modern medicine itself has become extremely specialized. It is divided into separate fields where uniform treatment regimes are applied to patients based on scientific, objective diagnosis of a disease. Drug therapy is at the forefront of this approach to treatment. Patients diagnosed with the "same" condition are given standardized, usually synthesized, chemical compounds. Only the frequency and concentration of the dosage varies between individuals. I once read that the best outcome for patients would be to dump all the pills into the ocean, although it would likely result in the worst outcome for marine life. By contrast, Oriental medicine may apply very different treatment approaches to patients, even when they outwardly exhibit the same or similar symptoms.

It seems that much of the focus and direction of modern Western medicine is under the control of pharmaceutical companies. They increasingly dictate the treatments available to doctors for their patients. Those losing out in this situation appear to be the patients, whose choices are severely limited. Western medicine developed much of its considerable expertise in emergency care and surgical intervention on the battlefield. Its effectiveness in acute situations, requiring intensive emergency care, is well proven. What it lacks is the means to handle the plague of increasingly chronic conditions that have arisen over the latter part of the twentieth century, and this situation continues to worsen in the new millennium. It would be in the best interests of human health if modern Western medicine accepted that there is no all-conquering medicine that can do everything. Acknowledging where its own strengths lie would allow it to welcome the participation of other complementary systems, such as Oriental medicine and therapies like shiatsu, to deal with the areas where it is ill-equipped. This could then result in a truly integrated health-care system, one where general practitioners are able to provide ki and tsubo treatment for their patients. Just as importantly, ordinary people would also have the means to offer basic healing through shiatsu to support the health and well-being of one another. There is real value in this for everyone, particularly for families, as it can also enhance relationships. This is truly something to be hoped for and worked toward: a world where we may once again see medicine that is centered on the human hand, with the power to heal residing not just with corporations and professionals, but with ordinary people.

HOW TO FIND TSUBO

Let us begin the practice that can make such a situation a reality. If at this stage you don't feel ready to begin, then please skip this practice section for now. However, I think you will find it very interesting. Try to be relaxed and not to feel that "you" have to be responsible to "do" something, as this creates tension and a feeling of heaviness. The best way to approach this practice is with childlike curiosity and a sense of humor. Don't be too serious. Find a friend or willing partner and ask if you can practice with them and borrow their arm. They will be referred to as the "receiver" and you—the person practicing the method—as the "giver." On the outside of the forearm below the elbow is a good area to begin working (see overleaf).

FINDING TSUBO IN A SELECTED AREA

1. Look at this area of the arm and imagine where the receiver most wants to be pressed.
2. Touch the point you imagined with your middle finger. You don't have to press hard, but with enough depth to reach between the skin and muscle. Keep trying to imagine how the receiver is feeling each moment as you press (this is the most important aspect!) and move your finger slightly back and forth.

If you can keep imagining how the receiver is feeling each moment (remember again that this is the purpose of what you are doing) you will become aware of a sensation that feels like the tip of a grain of rice, or a knot in a string. Its size can range from 1–3 mm, although it may sometimes be bigger.

Ask the receiver if they can feel the rice tip, as it is usually easier for the receiver to feel it before the giver. The sensation is not a superficial one. Some degree of depth of pressure by the giver is required for the receiver to feel the rice tip. Keep checking and confirming with the receiver until you find this depth. The receiver may experience a sense of fullness or pain, but it shouldn't be too uncomfortable. If it is not clear, return to the first step and look again.

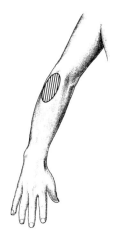

Finding tsubo on the outside of the forearm below the elbow.

The first step is cleared once you can feel the rice tip and the receiver confirms it.

Touch the tsubo with the center finger.

You must imagine where the receiver most wants to be pressed, rather than where *you* feel they want to be pressed. It has to be from the receiver's side. The place you imagine exists at once as the subject (in your imagination), but at the same time it is the object (the place the receiver wants to be pressed). This demonstrates a fundamental ki principle: the synchronization of subject and object. By imagining the point where the receiver most wants to be pressed, one of the many tsubo in that area will respond. Of course there are more than just one tsubo in the area. Also, if different people were to select the location on the same receiver by imagining the point most needing to be pressed, different tsubo would likely be chosen. This results from the differing capacity, or "depth," of each individual's empathetic imagination in identifying with, and caring for, the receiver's life. Each tsubo has a different location in the physical body and depth in the ki body. As the depth and strength of your empathetic imagination improves, so too does the capacity to connect to deeper tsubo. If you take one tsubo at a certain depth and treat it, other tsubo at a shallower depth around it will be treated simultaneously.

Unfortunately, I have no way to answer if your response to this experience is, "Why is this?" Can you simply try to accept the providence of nature at work?

FEELING THE ECHO OF THE TSUBO

The echo is a sensation of fullness, numbness, or an electric current-like traveling pain felt by the receiver when the tsubo, or rice tip, is pressed. The echo signals that stuck or stagnated ki, whose nature has become negative and dysfunctional, is being released. This stagnated ki is called *jaki*. It is the opposite of *seiki*, the life-sustaining energy whose unimpeded circulation is the basis of good health. The object of tsubo treatment in Tao Shiatsu is to release jaki from the body or transform it to seiki. Jaki is discussed in more detail in chapter three.

Three types of echo

1. **TO THE LIMBS AND HEAD.** The most common type of echo is from the tsubo location toward the extremities, i.e. the hands, feet, or head. Receiving shiatsu to a tsubo in the neck, for example, may create an echo in the arm or hand as jaki is released through the end points.

2. **TO THE TORSO.** The echo is sometimes felt from the torso toward the location being pressed. For example, when pressing a tsubo in the arm the echo is felt in the chest, signifying that the jaki in the chest is moving out. As treatment proceeds, the echo is likely to change and move toward the extremities, with the receiver then feeling it in the arm or hand.

3. **TO DEEP INSIDE.** An echo deep inside the tsubo (toward the body's core) occurs when jaki is very deeply located. There may be a sense of the echo reaching other parts of the body, but the strongest sensation is deep inside. Treatment will see the echo change to the pattern described in 1. or 2. above. This signifies that jaki deep inside is beginning to come to the surface, from where it can be released to the extremities.

In cases where jaki is too deep there may be no echo at all, just a superficial feeling in response to pressure. In this case the tsubo is closed. Choose another tsubo in the area. If no open tsubo can be found in an area, then choose another area. Alternatively, the reason for the lack of response could be that the giver is not touching the rice tip clearly, or is pressing physically without empathetic imagination.

FEELING THE ECHO OF THE TSUBO

1. Locate the tsubo with the middle finger and then press with the thumb for not more than 2-3 seconds.
2. Ask the receiver if they feel any echo and where it is felt.

At this point you have completed the preparation stage: locating the tsubo, feeling the rice tip, and confirming that there is an echo. Before you can actually give treatment by pressing the tsubo, you must clearly understand the way to apply pressure.

HOW TO PRESS TSUBO

Do the words "how to press the tsubo" make you think of physical technique, the form of the hand, or degree of pressure to apply? The ki world is the inner world of the heart and the outer material world synchronized as one. The tsubo must be pressed in a way that conforms to this principle of ki for treatment to be effective. Tao Shiatsu is not about the form of the hand. It is the development of the Tao heart—the heart of nature. This is what creates the effectiveness in shiatsu treatment. Directly experiencing the difference in response created by the change in the heart state in the following practice, is the only way to understand this.

PRESSING THE TSUBO

Locate a tsubo in the same area on the arm. Press it in the ways described in 1 and 2 below and after each, ask the receiver about the sensation created in both their heart and body.

1. Touch the tsubo (the sensation of the rice tip) and imagine it as only a part of the body. Apply continuous pressure for 2–3 seconds only. Now ask the receiver how it felt.
2. Touch the tsubo while continuously imagining that the receiver's whole body is included in this point. Press while continuously deepening this image. Try not to let the sense arise of the tsubo as only one part of the body. Continue for 2–3 seconds and then ask the receiver how it felt.

Now ask your partner what difference they could feel between the two ways. The experience of pressure in 1 is usually, to some degree, uncomfortable. In 2, if the image is maintained, a deep sense of comfort can be felt in the whole body.

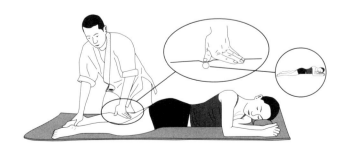

The tsubo includes the whole body.

As mentioned earlier, tsubo are a "double-edged sword." They are the gateways that enable deep and effective treatment of the meridians. Conversely, they are also the most vulnerable part of a person. The ki body can be injured if the tsubo is pressed without imagining it includes the whole body. The Austrian philosopher Rudolf Steiner (1861–1925) referred to the energy lines flowing in the ethereal body, or ki body, as it is known in Tao Shiatsu. The ki body surrounds the physical body extending in all directions up to a distance of two meters. The harm caused by mere physical pressure to the tsubo is often not apparent to the receiver at the time. There is often just a sensation of discomfort, and a symptom may even appear to go away with this kind of shiatsu. The effect is only temporary, however, as the symptom goes deeper inside the ki body and can re-emerge with increased intensity.

Before proceeding to treatment of the tsubo, further explanation is needed about the meridian system and the relationship of tsubo, jaki, and the kyo meridian to one another.

THE MERIDIANS AND THE KI FUNCTIONS THEY FACILITATE

Traditionally, twelve meridians and the extra meridians, known as the Conception and Governor Vessels, have been conceived of in Oriental medicine as making up the human energy system. People often misinterpret the meridians as being linked to particular anatomical organs because the names correspond, such as Lung, or Large Intestine. This is not the case. The meridians are not physical elements of the body. The use in Japan of equivalent names as the internal organs only came about during the Meiji period (1868–1912) when Western anatomy was introduced, and the meridian names were equated with the internal organs in order to translate these new and unfamiliar terms.

Single-cell life forms do not require the separation of the functions of their life activity. Amoebae have no need for multiple roles, so there is no requirement for a complex meridian system. Their locomotion by means of solgel movement exhibits the most holistic kyo and jitsu action. From the liquid state of solution (kyo), the amoebae tense through gelation (jitsu) causing a temporary protrusion. This is used as a foothold for motion, and propulsion is generated as the form relaxes and returns to solution once more. Master Masunaga described the kyo–jitsu pattern of amoebae as revealing the most basic mechanism of meridian function.

In the case of multiple-cell organisms, segmentation generates more cells. The permeation between cell walls creates a continuous exchange between the cells. As an organism becomes more complicated, its needs

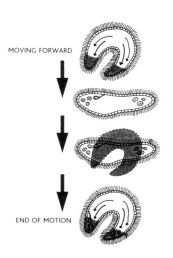

The solgel movement of amoebae.

require more than one cell to share the roles. In human beings this necessitates multiple meridians. A holistic approach to life requires that heart and body work together to bring about all activity. The twelve meridians form six pairs that facilitate the following life functions.

Lung and Large Intestine
Absorb external ki, exchange it, and eliminate the waste products.

Stomach and Spleen
Ingest and digest food to release its ki.

Heart and Small Intestine
Integrate and convert ki released in digestion.

Kidney and Bladder
Maintain vitality and purify the absorbed ki.

Heart Constrictor and Triple Heater
Circulate ki to the whole body and protect the borders.

Liver and Gallbladder
Store and distribute ki for practical activity.

Conception Vessel and Governor Vessel are extra meridians used in treatment. They play the role of a bypass when there is poor circulation in the twelve meridians.

NOTE: ki here refers to both heavenly ki such as air, and earth ki in the form of food and water.

The classics describe twelve meridians plus the two extra meridians. None of the meridians are shown flowing throughout the entire body. Six meridians—Lung and Large Intestine, Heart and Small Intestine, Heart Constrictor and Triple Heater—are not shown in the legs. The remaining six meridians—Stomach and Spleen, Kidney and Bladder, Liver and Gallbladder—are not shown in the arms. Master Masunaga was the first to seriously question whether this situation was satisfactory to provide effective treatment in modern times. Evidenced by the recent phenomenon in China of "new" acupuncture tsubo appearing every year, obviously it is not. Master Masunaga explained that the classical meridian chart showed only six of the twelve meridians in the arms, and the other six in the legs, because the movement toward mass education in acupuncture was well advanced by the time they were being written. Hence the meridian system was simplified for safety and convenience. Master Masunaga realized the existence of twelve meridians throughout the whole body by discovering that each meridian flowed in both the arms and legs.

Tao Shiatsu recognizes twenty-four meridians throughout the body. My clinical practice led to the identification of a sub-meridian belonging to each of the twelve whole-body meridians of Master Masunaga. Additionally, each of the twelve main meridians (as Tao Shiatsu describes them) has ring and spiral streams. This is a picture of the human meridian stream that seems to more closely resemble the holistic nature of the body. The process of discovery of the meridian world has been a long one. At times it has been an arduous journey to break through the walls of dogma that surround the classics. It has brought me to the understanding that tsubo are the fundamental expression of life. They exist only on the meridian that is kyo, or deficient in energy. By its nature, which is emptiness, the fundamental impulse of kyo is to be filled with ki. This takes place when it is able to unify with the universal ki, as occurs during shiatsu treatment. Only one meridian can exist as the specific kyo meridian at any given moment. When we fully recognize that the main and extra meridians are streaming with sub, ring, and spiral branches, we see the many possible locations where tsubo may appear on the meridian that is kyo.

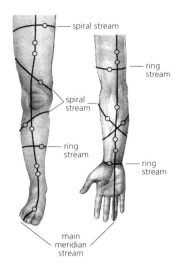

Tsubo may be located on any or all of the kyo meridian's streams.

UNDERSTANDING THE CAUSE OF KYO AND JITSU MERIDIANS

Kyo is usually explained in books on Oriental medicine as the meridian, relative to all the other meridians, in which there is a deficiency or dispersal of ki. Jitsu, on the other hand, is described as the meridian in which there is a relative excess or concentration of ki. This description is not wholly satisfactory, however, because it does not address what brings about the imbalance of ki in the meridians. A deeper understanding of kyo and its relationship to jaki—stuck or stagnated ki—needs to be addressed. The Japanese word *kyo* comes from the Chinese word *koku* meaning emptiness: empty, but never in the sense of lifeless, for this is the Source of Life itself. The great Taoist philosophers Lao Tsu (6th century B.C.) and Sun Tzu (c. 500 B.C.) described the heart of the universe as the "world of emptiness" that inherently wishes to be filled. Tao, The Great Void, Infinite Nature—whatever name we call it by, the kyo meridian is connected to it.

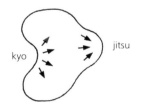

The relationship of kyo and jitsu.

Tsubo only exist on the kyo meridian, so treating them discharges jaki

Tsubo are the access points to connect to jaki: pressing tsubo discharges jaki through the echo. All disease is created by jaki. It creates the distortion of the meridian and the resulting kyo and jitsu pattern which gives rise to adverse symptoms. For example, if there is neck pain, there will be tsubo in that area: pressing them will cause an echo that may be deep inside, or down into the arm and then the fingertips. Locating and treating tsubo in the area of pain until the echo changes or lessens will relieve the symptom.

No standard theory about jaki exists in Oriental medicine. The kanji for *ja* in jaki (邪気) comes from the original Chinese character that represents something that does not fit. In terms of the human energy system, jaki forms as stuck or stagnated ki that burdens and impedes meridian circulation. Imbalance and disharmony is expressed through the symptoms of the kyo–jitsu meridian pattern. From the point of view of meridian treatment, the kyo meridian is the ki stream that is most strongly trying to discharge jaki. There is a natural law at work as our body attempts to neutralize or discharge anything negative or harmful that enters. Consider what happens when you eat something that is contaminated by unhealthy bacteria: the digestive system will attempt to expel it through vomiting or diarrhea. This mechanism functions not only physiologically. At all levels of life, from the heart to ki and meridians, the impulse exists to expel jaki. This natural law of discharge operates as the kyo meridian stimulates the jitsu meridian to activity that will accomplish this. All symptoms of the mind and body—pain, injury, stress, tension, anxiety, and desire—express the attempt to discharge jaki. They all seek expression through activity that provides release. In the terms of a most fundamental aspect of Oriental philosophy, yin and yang, the symptoms are the manifestation of the yang impulse arising. Yin and yang are the two mutually contradictory properties of all phenomena and share a simultaneous cause and effect relationship. Western medicine tends to focus on the symptoms—the external expression of the deeper yin aspect—as the problem to be fixed or eradicated. The real source of each person's symptoms, though, is the attempt by the individual's life force to release jaki, thus ensuring it does not become excessively burdened or overwhelmed by it.

ACCESSING THE KYO MERIDIAN

Just as each individual has a heart, so does the universe. This is sometimes described as the essence of Greater Nature. The perception of distance and space are created by our consciousness. In the ki world there is no distance. What exists is the state of infinite spreading, or expansion. This is not merely philosophy: astronomy has revealed that the universe is in a state of constant expansion. This can be experienced through pressing the kyo meridian. The receiver feels their whole body subconsciously relax:

there is no distance or boundaries; just the sensation of infinite spreading, that provides the deepest sense of relief. Only through the kyo meridian is it experienced. Through pressing and reaching the bottom of the kyo meridian, jaki is released to the Greater Nature and seiki is able to replenish the deficiency. The "bottom" is the depth at which the receiver feels this response. It is the depth subconsciously felt by the receiver in their heart through the depth of the giver's empathetic imagination, synchronized with the depth reached in the ki body and the depth of pressure in the physical body. To allow the receiver to experience the relaxation response, the kyo line—the line through which the kyo meridian is accessed—has to be located. Previously the tsubo location was found with the method of using an image (where the receiver most wants to be pressed). To now locate the kyo line, a different method is used, which focuses on saying aloud the word "kyo."

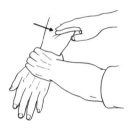

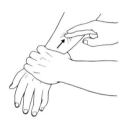

LOCATING THE KYO LINE

1. Return to the forearm area of the receiver. Empty your mind of any thoughts or doubts, and say out loud the word "kyo." While maintaining the image of the word, slide your middle finger across the forearm toward you. Try to resist any feeling of "trying to find" the kyo line.
2. Your finger will naturally stop.
3. The kyo line is the line through which the kyo meridian can be accessed. Imagine how the receiver subconsciously feels each moment and press this line with the middle finger to some degree of depth. Ask the receiver how it feels.
4. If the line and depth are right, the receiver will feel the relaxation response. If it is not clear, repeat steps 1–3.

Demonstrating this way of working usually provokes a torrent of questions, especially when teaching seminars and workshops in the West. Since I have now grown accustomed to this, let me attempt to explain what is happening. Ki responds to both the image and the word, so if the finger's movement is synchronized with the word it will stop naturally. However, just because the finger stops at a location corresponding to a line on the meridian chart, it does not necessarily mean that this is the kyo meridian. The receiver might be, for example, Large Intestine kyo, but the finger does not stop at the place shown as Large Intestine on the meridian chart. Yet the receiver feels the whole body relax when this line is pressed. Naturally this creates much confusion for students who observe it, especially the first time. A basic misunderstanding about the existence of the meridians is the source of this confusion.

Meridians are commonly understood to exist on or near the surface of the physical body. The classics explain the meridians as flowing in the spaces between the muscles. However, the meridian chart is merely a two-dimensional representation. It depicts the position where the meridian can be most easily accessed. This occurs because the meridian "comes up" toward the surface when the body is moved into a particular position, or the limbs stretched in a particular direction. With the body in another position, the meridian will exist more deeply in the ki body, up to a depth of about two meters. The meridians exist well beyond the limits of the physical body. The physical body can in fact be understood as the shadow of the ki body. The place you touch on the physical body (as shown on the chart) is just the location that, combined with the best angle or direction of pressure, will most clearly connect to the meridian in the ki body. The meridian chart must be understood as revealing the body position and surface location to access the meridians with perpendicular pressure. Changing the receiver's body position even slightly will change the access location and angle to that meridian. This surface access area on the physical body may shift by a range of up to five centimeters. If the meridian chart is not clearly understood as representing the access lines with the body in precisely that position, then this confusion will always arise.

So just say the word "kyo" and slide your finger until it naturally stops. The kyo meridian can be accessed if you put your entire effort toward keeping and increasing empathetic imagination for the receiver. This is possible without any prior knowledge of the meridians or needing to consult the meridian chart.

Some people, especially those with previous knowledge of the meridians, will still ask, "How can this be? What is it all about?" Even before attempting to experience it directly, there is doubt and scepticism. This is the conscious ego resisting. It is not easy for the ego to accept that the subconscious "knows" where to access the kyo, what angle to press, and the best depth. The world of ki is the world of the subconscious. The conscious ego drives the feeling of "trying to find" or "doubting what is found," which suppresses the wisdom of the subconscious. The starting point of this way of recognizing and treating the meridians is to accept that you must give up reliance on the ego and its dependence on conscious knowledge and information. As the giver's conscious ego recedes, the receiver's ki and subconscious will appear more clearly. The ego can only disturb and interrupt what is required to holistically activate the subconscious. Even though it is an essential part of daily living, it cannot help you in any way in the practice of shiatsu. Giving up dependence on the conscious ego will allow the ki world to reveal itself. To begin with, however, this is very difficult for our ego to accept.

Locating the tsubo of the kyo meridian is only possible with empathetic imagination

Clearly understanding the real nature of tsubo and the kyo meridian opens the door to the next stage. The receiver's ki responds each moment to the heart state and mental attitude of the giver. This was demonstrated in the earlier practice when the giver located the tsubo by imagining where the receiver most wanted to be pressed, which encouraged ki to react and the tsubo location to reveal itself.

The reason why the tsubo that was "taken" with empathetic imagination did not equate with the position on the meridian chart of the diagnosed meridian became clear to me only after many years of research. As noted earlier, the classics describe twelve major meridians, with six of these meridians streaming in the arms and six in the legs. Master Masunaga's research revealed the twelve meridians streaming in all the limbs. Tao Shiatsu has identified the existence of twelve additional sub-meridians. Each sub-meridian is related to one of the twelve main meridians and, like them, stream in all of the limbs, hence there are twenty-four whole-body meridians. Additional branches of each meridian are the ring and spiral streams. With each meridian encompassing the whole body, the locations for taking tsubo on the kyo meridian go far beyond the places revealed in the classical meridian chart. This means that really locating and connecting to tsubo of the kyo meridian can only be guaranteed through empathetic imagination.

Lung meridian—main and sub line on the hand.

The part includes the whole

Earlier in this chapter, I described how to press the tsubo while maintaining an image of it including the whole body. This is in complete accordance with Oriental philosophy's most fundamental principle—that the whole exists in each and every part. It is an understanding that has shaped all of the cultural and social forms of the East, including medicine. Only repeatedly and directly experiencing this at the level of the heart state makes it possible to comprehend what the head alone can never realize. That the whole is included in each and every part is one of the foundations of Eastern thinking. In shiatsu therapy and training, the shiatsu method, along with the words and images that express it, must be unified with this philosophy.

The bottom of the tsubo

Tsubo treatment is only effective because each tsubo includes the whole body and is thus able to affect it. Every tsubo has a different depth in the ki body, and to give effective shiatsu you must reach the bottom of this depth in the ki body. With tsubo existing only on the kyo meridian, the receiver feels the whole body relax when they are pressed with empathetic imagination. This allows the bottom of the tsubo to be reached and jaki to be released. If shiatsu fails to reach the bottom depth, ki cannot affect the whole body, though the receiver may still experience the relaxation response. Therefore it is vital for the shiatsu's depth to reach the bottom of the tsubo.

The receiver subconsciously feels the bottom of the tsubo as the bottom depth of their whole body, which includes the ki body. This sensation is one of absolute satisfaction and of something completely fitting. Again, it must be pointed out that the tsubo's depth cannot be simply understood as a physical depth in the body: it is at once the depth seen in the heart, the depth imagined in the ki body, and the physical depth of the thumb. The depth of the heart is simultaneously that of giver and receiver, because working with deep empathetic imagination creates heart unity. The giver's consciousness will never be able to determine this depth. For the beginner this is not something that can be judged, but it is possible to develop the capacity to feel the bottom by developing empathetic imagination.

KI IS CHANGING EACH MOMENT

The world we live in exists as an ever-changing stream of ki. Much research in quantum physics is confirming this, and conclusions presented in writings such as Fritjof Capra's *The Tao of Physics* support what Oriental philosophy has expressed for thousands of years, if not as lyrically and poetically. The full realization of Einstein's formulation, that energy and matter are completely interchangeable entities, is yet to fully manifest itself in humanity's day-to-day approach to living. This is particularly true in the West, where a stronger tendency remains to perceive things in fixed, concrete terms, with the material world very much the central focus. Thus the words "bottom of the tsubo" typically prompt people to imagine it as a particular physical depth.

Just as life is changing every moment, so too is the depth of the tsubo. When the tsubo is pressed with the image that it includes the whole body, the receiver feels very comfortable. After a few seconds, however, it is common for this to change, and it begins to feel uncomfortable. What is happening is that after the empathetic depth of the giver's shiatsu reaches the bottom of the tsubo, the receiver's ki responds by spreading throughout the ki body. It then attempts to release itself back to the universal ki of

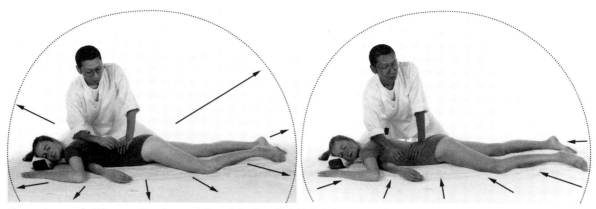

The receiver can feel the sensation change at the point where their ki starts to come up to the surface.

nature. Pushing back against the giver's pressure is the way it does this. It signals that the bottom of the tsubo is coming up and the depth is now shallower. This is a very delicate sensation. If the giver does not feel this response and continues to press, ki is prevented from being released. There is nowhere else for it to go but return inside where it may cause harm to the ki body, as evidenced by the discomfort felt by the receiver.

Usually the receiver can feel the sensation change at the point where their ki starts to come up to the surface. Often this sensation is described as "feeling enough." It occurs when ki reaches the border of the ki body, and its natural impulse at this point is to come back up to the surface to be released. Especially in the beginning of tsubo training, it is essential you always ask the receiver to indicate when this point is reached. Always try to adapt every moment to the receiver's responding ki—this is a fundamental principle of treating tsubo.

UNDERSTANDING THE MEANING OF TSUBO PRACTICE

"Imagine how the receiver is feeling each and every moment." It is easy to say these words, just as it was to describe the principle of tsubo location: "Imagine where the receiver most wants to be pressed." In reality you must forget about yourself in order to be able to see the receiver's heart and connect with their ki, their very life-sensation. As you should now be more aware, this is no easy task for your ego. Imagining how the receiver feels should not be restricted to the practice of shiatsu alone: it is the foundation of the human heart. Expressing it beyond the dojo (place of study) and the clinic is the real meaning of "practice." Giving your life to doing the best for others is itself the purpose, and being able to see and treat the tsubo is simply what results from this. It is not the goal of this training. The key to empathetic imagination is to care for others without distraction or loss of concentration. When this heart state is unified with the shiatsu method, or rather when it *becomes* the shiatsu method, ki will be able to naturally respond and come to the surface, release itself to the ki of nature, and discharge jaki. Naturally the conscious ego will fight and resist this loss of inward attention toward it. To begin with it is difficult to synchronize the shiatsu method and empathetic imagination, so you need to ask and confirm with the receiver while practicing. Devotion to this training will deepen the receiver's well-being from your shiatsu.

It is very easy to respond to the instruction "Every moment continuously imagine how the receiver is feeling" as just words. Sometimes people counter that if your heart is the subject of your imagination, it would seem to be the opposite of seeing the ki state of another person. However, actually experiencing this directly through empathetic imagination makes you realize that in fact the two unify and become one. This is the way to experience the universal heart that reveals ki. The moment-to-moment changes in the movement of ki become clear when the sense of self is diminished.

This may seem like a lot to practice, but realizing that this is the only way to release ki by tsubo treatment is the start. Practice without giving in to the conscious ego. Your imagination will begin to deepen to a point where there is complete oneness with the receiver's ki, when the hearts of giver and receiver reflect each other like mirrors.

THE TSUBO METHOD

Return to the outside of the forearm on the other arm as shown in first photo on the following page.

1. Locate the tsubo with empathetic imagination and check the rice tip with the middle finger.
2. Press the rice tip with the thumb. Ask and confirm if there is an echo.
3. Deepen empathetic imagination and let the pressure of the thumb follow until the receiver tells you that the shiatsu is reaching the bottom of the tsubo.
4. After a second or two, the bottom of the tsubo begins to push back. Try to feel this sensation, but only through increasing empathetic imagination. Always ask the receiver to tell you when they feel it is enough.
5. Adapt your shiatsu to the ki response, by synchronizing imagination and movement as you come up to the surface.

Locate another tsubo with empathetic imagination and repeat steps 1 to 5.

After treating a number of tsubo in an area, the strength of the echo will decrease as jaki is discharged. Move to the next area. Practicing on the limbs minimizes the effect of incorrect treatment, so only practice on the arms and legs at first. Only when all steps of the method are clearly experienced and confirmed by the receiver should you move to another area of the body.

Practice on the outside of the lower leg, below the knee, as shown in the second photo below, then practice with the other areas illustrated.

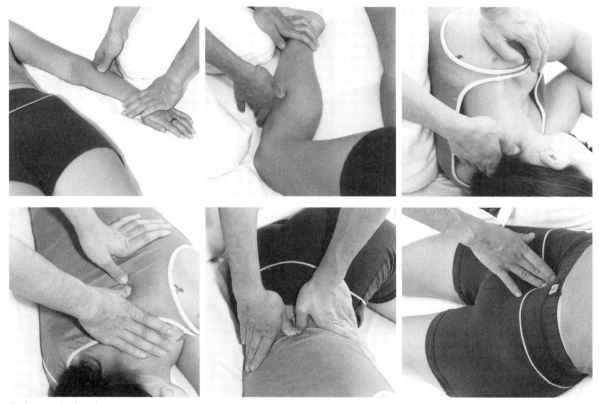

Tsubo practice locations.
Above: forearm, lower leg, neck.   Below: shoulder, waist, abdomen.

EXPRESSING THE HEART OF SHIATSU

Shiatsu is one of the best basic therapies for life. It is central to all Oriental medical practice. The response to pressure is the most fundamental manifestation of life and can be witnessed at all levels of existence. Witness how energy is exchanged between cells by the mechanism of homeostatic pressure, allowing them to pass their contents to one another, or how atmospheric pressure produces the winds that spread seeds and pollen to assist plants and trees to reproduce.

Shiatsu is pressure that is changing every moment, a flexible adaption to heart and ki. When a true master practices acupuncture, the location and depth of each needle's insertion should be determined by looking at the response of the whole body. Similarly, doctors of Chinese herbal medicine determine the diagnosis and corresponding dosage by adapting to the patient's ki. The human hand when put in the service of the heart is ideally suited to medical treatment. Shiatsu and other manual therapies are at the core of Oriental medicine for this reason. Tools or substances themselves can only be guided and administered by adapting through the heart to the moment-by-moment changes in ki.

Oriental medicine often speaks philosophically of the sage as the "ideal person," but not in the same sense as the saint in Western terms. Such a person may seem to belong to another dimension, removed from everyday life. Yet the oneness of heart and action of the sage is the real message their life gives us. Western thought evolved to realize matter as separate from consciousness, yet our bodies fully express and are the expression of our hearts. Equally, our societies or communities are the collective expression of all those who live in them. While there is so much preoccupation in the modern world with the external influences of good health, such as exercise, diet, and health supplements, what is really necessary for optimal health is the attitude of the heart. Living and acting through the heart for the well-being of others is the basic way to a healthy body. Medicine must always show the way toward this and reflect the image of the ideal human being. The heart of the saints and sages is not an unattainable ideal; it is the flexible adaptation of ki to the constant change of life. This should be the aim of a healthy lifestyle. In the setting of the shiatsu clinic, it is the completely flexible adaptation to the patient's ki and assisting it to adapt to the constant change in the whole of nature. Each tsubo includes the whole body. The whole of nature is present in each and every individual human heart and body. These are the secrets of the unity of the ki world.

3

THE DEPTHS OF THE KI WORLD

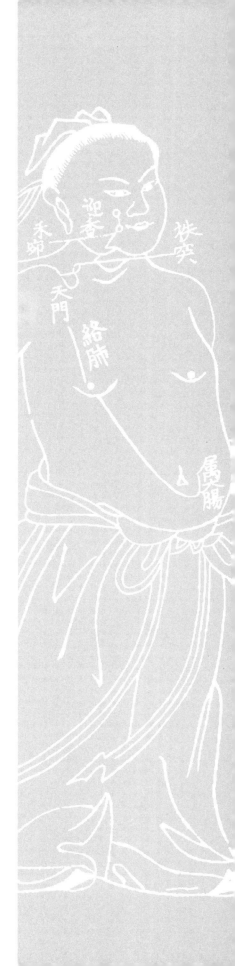

Eight Stages toward the Internalized Distortion of Ki

FIRST STAGE
SEEING AND LOCATING TSUBO

Tsubo are the starting point of the journey into the ki world. The first step in tsubo shiatsu—"imagine the point where the receiver most wants to be pressed"—opens the gateway. Generally, at the first stage people are unable to see ki. The previous chapter shows how this starts to become possible. For the student who wishes to step through this gateway, two things are necessary. The tsubo must be found with empathy and imagination and the receiver's life sensation must be continuously felt at each moment through the tsubo. This process reveals the location, and eventually also the size and bottom depth of the tsubo. As the empathetic imagination of the giver develops, the bottom of the tsubo is felt coming up and then pushing back against the thumb. Finally the tsubo disappears as it fills with ki. Doubts about the existence of tsubo also disappear with this experience, as does the concept of tsubo as named and numbered fixed points. Shiatsu has no need to be tied to this interpretation of tsubo as acupuncture points, derived from the classics.

Experience the real nature of tsubo as described in the previous chapter and step into the first stage of the ki world. At this point the subject (giver's imagination) and the object (receiver's tsubo) are not completely one. The location of the tsubo appears to exist objectively, that is, outside the giver. However, only by synchronizing the object as the subject of the imagination does the tsubo in fact exist for the giver. The degree of separation that remains between subject and object is what causes the tsubo and its bottom depth in the ki body to be unclear. In this, the preparation stage, the student's heart is poised on standby. What is crucial in moving forward is to resist seeking "results," such as "trying to find the tsubo." Instead put all your effort toward seeing what creates the separation. Try to clearly realize how the "self-sensation" that is constantly arising is inhibiting empathetic imagination of the receiver's life-sensation. This will only disappear with continuous effort toward an egoless heart. Follow this process each time you are locating the tsubo and adapting shiatsu to the responding ki.

SECOND STAGE
SEEING KI SPREADING

Continuous practice of the first stage of tsubo shiatsu leads in time to the ability to visualize ki. Seeing ki spread is the subject of the second stage.

Three points can summarize tsubo shiatsu thus far:

1. Imagine that the tsubo includes the whole body and retain this image while pressing.

2. Reach the bottom of the tsubo through deep empathy toward the receiver's life-sensation.

3. Adapt your shiatsu to the receiver's constantly changing ki, which includes the tsubo's bottom depth, by continuously deepening empathetic imagination.

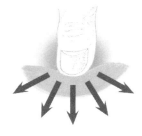

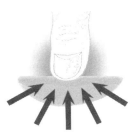

When the bottom of the tsubo is reached, it tries to come up to the surface.

Space and time are dimensions with an inseparable relationship in the Tsubo Method. The tsubo including the receiver's whole body is the spatial aspect, while the moment-to-moment adaptation to the receiver's ki is the temporal aspect. What image do the words "the tsubo includes the whole body" create for you? Is it one where the body is a fixed and unchanging form? In reality our bodies are constantly changing, much more like a liquid than a solid. When the bottom of the tsubo is reached, it tries to come up to the surface. It is changing every moment just like the whole body it includes. Like a photograph capturing a moment, the "body" that is consciously recognized in daily life is only a part of the whole. The whole is always flexible, everchanging and incapable of being recognized through conscious thought. So our conscious grasp on life is limited in relation to that of the subconscious, much like the visible tip of an iceberg represents only a small part of its entire mass. Life equals ki: both exist as an everchanging stream. The conscious world is a part of the whole but it is not the whole. To affect the whole body you must constantly recognize it as everchanging, then it becomes easier to press the tsubo and imagine it including the whole body.

Principles of tsubo treatment

In practice and treatment always try to:

1. Keep imagining how the receiver feels.

2. Ask about the depth and timing of pressure.

3. Adapt flexibly to the responding ki so that you begin to release pressure and come up to the surface before the receiver says "enough."

Experiencing the steps of tsubo treatment

Through continuous empathetic imagination the following stages are recognized:

1. The rice tip (tsubo).

2. The bottom depth of the tsubo.

3. The adaptation response (the receiver's ki pressing back against the giver's thumb).

Tsubo shiatsu is effective and comfortable for the receiver when these principles and steps are followed. Practicing the method consistently allows the image and action to begin to enter into the subconscious. From this point, synchronizing image and method becomes a more natural response, requiring less and less conscious direction. As this occurs, what you are seeing will change. The receiver's ki begins to appear, responding to the continuous pressure applied with empathetic imagination. When this process penetrates the subconscious, the giver's shiatsu and receiver's ki become one, making it possible to see the response of ki to pressure. The phenomenon of ki spreading can be clearly experienced when giving shiatsu to the *hara*—the abdomen. All of the meridians pass through this region and have specific diagnostic areas identified by Master Masunaga. Applying four-finger pressure with empathetic imagination to these diagnostic areas causes ki to spread with a different response pattern for each meridian. The kyo meridian can be identified because of its unique response pattern, whereby ki spreads to the whole body. The ranges with which ki spreads in the other meridians are limited in comparison to the kyo meridian, and do not reach the whole body. When the giver presses a kyo meridian that exists in the lower abdomen, the whole-body feeling is experienced very clearly. Jitsu (excess of ki) symptoms will disappear, while a kyo (deficiency of ki) symptom will lessen but not disappear completely. In cases where a kyo meridian exists in the upper abdomen, the situation is slightly different. Pressing a kyo meridian here creates the feeling of "finding the missing piece in a puzzle." These responses are the subconscious feeling of the receiver and not that of the giver's touch sense. Only by the giver deepening empathetic imagination can the receiver's subconscious clearly experience these responses.

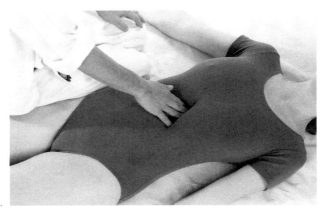

Four finger pressure to the hara meridian.

Awakening the primal sense

A heightened primal sense still exists in those who live in a close relationship with nature and the land, such as Bushmen and other indigenous peoples. The toxins produced by modern living have not invaded their spirit, hence they are able to naturally forecast the following day's weather, communicate with spirits, and see past lives. This is commonly referred to as the intuitive sense and is possessed by everyone. Shamans are those whose primal sense is especially developed. These ancient abilities have become considerably weakened in the majority of modern people, especially city dwellers. Let us consider a simple example that many people may be familiar with in the context of the primal sense. It occurs sometimes when you spontaneously think about someone, then shortly afterward the telephone rings and they have called you. This is usually explained as "coincidence" or "chance," although the feeling that you experience of "just maybe it wasn't by chance" is the response of the primal sense. When this capacity is fully awakened in some people, often manifesting in what appear to be supernatural abilities, they can often mistake it as a form of spiritual enlightenment, as do people around them. This phenomenon is witnessed currently in the rise of individuals who promote themselves as New Age gurus. However, this is in no way related to the state of enlightenment that spiritual traditions such as Buddhism refer to. It is simply the awakening of the primal sense.

Keeping this caution in mind, let us return to tsubo shiatsu. Feeling the whole body respond, not a part of it, brings diagnosis one step closer. The basis of diagnosis is determining whether or not ki spreads in response to pressure. This opens the way to experiencing the whole body response that comes from pressing the kyo meridian. Of course this remains unclear at first, but little by little it starts to appear. The ancient Chinese referred to the receiver's ki response as *mei* (明), also translated as "light" and meaning "wisdom." Oriental medicine itself was perceived as "the light." Without this illumination and wisdom, knowledge of the meridian stream was considered superficial and therapy had to rely on the touch sense. In Oriental medical healing, this physical sense has to be surpassed. Traditionally, all Oriental doctors and physicians were trained through manual therapy to see ki and meridians. When it could be seen how ki responded and spread, diagnosis became possible. The most appropriate form of treatment could then be applied, be it via the hand (manual therapy), the needle (acupuncture), or a herbal remedy.

In shiatsu this means that the giver can clearly perceive ki responding when the tsubo or meridian is pressed. There is then no need to rely on the chart to connect to the meridian. This relieves the tension of trying to find the exact spot indicated by the meridian chart. Instead the judgment of location and depth is based on whether ki responds or not. Repeatedly practicing with empathetic imagination while constantly imagining that the tsubo includes the whole body leads to the opening of the subconscious and the ki world.

THIRD STAGE
BOSHIN—DIAGNOSING BY "LOOKING"

Boshin is Oriental medicine's term for diagnosis performed by only looking. This advanced level of diagnosis determines the situation of the meridians without any physical contact with the receiver's body. Facial diagnosis is described in the classics as an example of boshin. It is stated, for example, that the appearance of whiteness or very pale skin color of the face indicates a condition that relates to the Large Intestine and Lung meridians. Taking this literally, however, would imply that all people with this skin tone be diagnosed in the same way, so care needs to be taken in how we understand boshin.

When I first saw Master Masunaga diagnose simply by looking, I wondered how such a thing was possible. It seemed like the work of God, and felt very mysterious to witness. Later when I briefly lost the ability to diagnose in this way, I realized how hard it is to actually do. Boshin develops from the process that begins with recognizing tsubo and meridians, which is followed by the ability to adapt to the receiver's spirit and then see ki spread. The process of boshin was happening almost entirely in my subconscious and meant that I was unable to find the words to explain exactly how it was being done. What enabled me to gradually find a way to explain it were the regular workshops I began to teach in the West. The endless questions that were asked by students witnessing this form of diagnosis had to be answered in English, which is not my native language. This gave me a unique opportunity to look much more closely and try to find a way to describe this subconscious process. In shiatsu, sho diagnosis—determining the ki stimulation needed to return the receiver's life force to a holistic state—is performed through hara diagnosis, which reveals the kyo meridian in the abdomen. At any given time only one of the meridian streams in the hara is in a state of complete oneness with Greater Nature. By looking at the hara, I am able to visualize which meridian exhibits the state of "emptiness" and infinite spreading of ki. This is the basis of making an accurate diagnosis. As explained earlier, the kyo meridian is not empty in the sense of containing nothing, but empty in that it has the capacity to include everything.

Reaching the stage of boshin not only changes the way you look at the receiver's body; it also reverses what you see. Usually we see the physical body in close-up, as the material subject in the foreground. The surrounding space is perceived as the background. Looking at the same situation through boshin, the background (or Nature) that supports the whole becomes the subject. The receiver's body is recognized as a part of the whole, existing inside it. While there is actually no border between the body and the whole of Nature, we see it as separate when viewed with our daily-life consciousness. Initially, the range of your imagination in determining where the receiver most wants to be pressed is limited to imagining a specific area, such as the forearm. Once the level of boshin is reached, the imagination becomes much wider and able to encompass the whole body. What takes place is an expansion of the giver's spirit, reflected by a quantum leap in the capacity of the imagination. As human beings we depend on our physical eyes to see, so when we view the receiver's body, we are only able to see one part of it in any given moment. If we look at the hara, for example, we cannot physically see the receiver's back as well. It is impossible to see the whole with the material eye and the physical senses alone. If the imagination is concentrated deeply, however, then the whole body can be "viewed" at once from all angles. If the giver constantly practices by looking with the eyes, while simultaneously imagining the whole, the range of the imagination expands making it possible to "see" beyond the material level. Just like Nature, the receiver's ki is constantly changing. Flexibility of the giver's spirit enables the receiver's body to be viewed from all angles, revealing the constant change in the wholeness of the receiver. Since ki follows the image, it will begin to react and spread without any physical pressure from the fingers. The giver's image of pressing the meridian must be very strong and completely synchronized. By this mechanism it is possible to see each meridian's ki spreading, and diagnose only with the imagination.

This process can neither be performed nor understood consciously. Trying to picture it with your common sense may create the idea that it must take time, as the giver imagines pressing each of the meridians individually. However, when seeing through this heart state the dimension of time completely alters. I found that I could clearly recognize eighteen distinct intervals occurring in each second, almost as if time slowed down. So in a single second the response pattern of all the meridians can be seen and the kyo meridian identified. Realistically, though, in clinical practice a few seconds are required to confirm and ensure there is no mistake. Only by analyzing my subconscious have I been able to explain it in this way. The world of the heart and subconscious does not suddenly appear one day. Rather, it arises by constantly investigating where the receiver most wants to be pressed, locating the tsubo, then each moment imagining how they are feeling as you press. Sho diagnosis of the hara meridians only becomes possible when the ki body of giver and receiver unify and become one. The giver is then simply able to follow the receiver's life force as it freely expresses itself.

FOURTH STAGE
DIAGNOSING THE STIFFNESS OF THE KYO MERIDIAN

The path that revealed to me the stiffness of the kyo meridian followed years of checking my clinical experience with the gifts of Master Masunaga's books and teachings. In this way I was able to confirm my experiences. When I first began giving shiatsu, I could not perform accurate diagnosis by pressing the hara meridians and was unable to "see" the kyo meridian.

Until 1983 this did not pose much of a problem. Almost all patients receiving treatment exhibited jitsu symptoms, which presented in the body as pain or stiffness caused by the excessive concentration of ki. By pressing the meridian in the limbs which I felt to be kyo, I was able to reach the bottom of tsubo to dissipate the concentrated ki, relieving the pain or stiffness relatively easily. Giving a prescribed sequence of shiatsu for the whole body, known as Basic Form, preceded tsubo treatment. This combination proved effective in treating most patients.

Things began to change from 1985, when what I call the "time age" reached a turning point to bring about a situation where more than 90% of patients exhibited kyo rather than jitsu-type symptoms. Simply diagnosing and pressing the kyo meridian of the limbs was now no longer adequate. At first I was baffled and unsure what to do. However, by continuing the process of diagnosing the associated meridian and treating tsubo around the symptom area, the effectiveness of my treatments again increased and I began to understand what was happening. Deep inside the tsubo of the kyo meridian, I began to see a "stiffness" that existed at a previously unrecognized level.

The unity and oneness of the ki world is demonstrated at each stage: experiencing tsubo; seeing ki spread; the appearance of kyo through boshin; and now the kyo stiffness becoming visible. Absolute oneness of subject and object is beyond comparison and conflict. In this state the situation of the meridian is as clear as any object seen in daily life. Studying the meridian diagnosis system of Master Masunaga had greatly deepened my respect for him and his devotion to shiatsu. The signposts he provided directed my journey and greatly helped to confirm my own findings. Eventually, though, as my experiences moved beyond those discussed in his books, there was nothing left to refer to for confirmation. I was now proceeding alone, yet felt I had no other option but to continue.

Releasing the Energy Distortion Created by Jaki

FIFTH STAGE
DISCOVERING THE WHOLE-BODY MERIDIAN

The discovery of the kyo stiffness is one of Master Masunaga's legacies and it was this deeper state of ki that became the focus of my clinical practice and research. Great effectiveness in treating my patient's pain and symptoms resulted from the practice of meridian shiatsu, based on Masunaga's twelve whole body meridians and the two extra meridians. Then a puzzling pattern began to emerge. Some patients felt pain and revealed kyo stiffness—noticeably in the lower back and neck—which did not correspond with where my sho diagnosis of the kyo meridian in the hara would have predicted it to be. These cases were the first indication that the range of the meridian stream revealed by Master Masunaga's research alone was no longer sufficient to explain and treat the symptoms I was witnessing in my clinical practice. Master Masunaga himself would have no doubt confronted a similar situation in his clinical practice, prompting him to expand on the twelve classical acupuncture meridians.

For me this puzzle was to be solved as the presentation of the patients' symptoms changed fundamentally in the mid-1980s. I first treated an extremely rare case where the symptom was expressed not through the jitsu but the kyo meridian. Generally symptoms and pain were expressed through the jitsu (excess of ki) meridian. This meant treatment was given to the kyo (deficient in ki) meridian, but usually on the opposite side to where the pain was experienced. The rationale was that the kyo meridian existed "behind" the symptom; so excess ki was drawn to the deficiency, thus relieving the jitsu symptom. Now the kyo meridian presented itself in the "foreground." A shift in the human meridian and energetic system was taking place. The kyo had drawn deeper into the ki body, giving rise to symptoms on the kyo meridian itself. Instead of going from the main area of pain and treating the kyo meridian on the other side, I followed the sho diagnosis but treated the kyo stiffness in the kyo meridian stream that flowed "horizontally" (see left illustration below on the following page). My patient was amazed that the pain was relieved, although perhaps not as amazed as I was, wondering what this completely different way of practicing meridian shiatsu meant. I soon realized why increasing numbers of my patients' symptoms had not been relieved with the previous treatment approach.

This was the point in tsubo treatment where I experienced the kyo stiffness that Master Masunaga had described. Seeing and treating what existed deep inside the kyo meridian relieved my patients' pain and symptoms. However, a mystery still remained in that I was finding kyo stiffness in places that did not match where the diagnosed kyo meridian was shown to stream, even on the extended Zen Shiatsu chart. For example, one of my patients complained of neck pain. Sho diagnosis of her hara revealed Large Intestine kyo, which conventionally would lead me to look in the front of the neck where the Large Intestine meridian streamed (see right illustration below on the following page). Naturally I thought the symptom would exist there. To my surprise, however, the kyo stiffness presented itself on the back of the neck. I was able to treat the kyo stiffness but was confused and unable to explain this situation.

The mid-1980s heralded the "Kyo Age." I use this term to describe the overall deepening of the kyo state. Symptoms deepened and their presentation shifted from the jitsu to the kyo meridian. The ki response became increasingly shallow in many patients, making clinical practice much more challenging. In an increasing number of cases, treating and reaching the bottom depth of the correctly diagnosed kyo meridian in the limbs no longer relieved a patient's symptoms. Due to this overall deepening of the kyo state, the kyo meridian had become so internalized that it reached a depth where it was effectively "closed" to treatment. Giving shiatsu treatment to the meridian in this state is meaningless. Now I was left to ponder, "How could I give effective treatment in the Kyo Age?" The answer became clear only by concentrating my heart and trying to see the deeper ki level.

What I found was that, even when a kyo meridian becomes deeply internalized and closed, there still exists a meridian in which ki responds. It exists on the other side of the limb, neck, or torso, in a symmetrical relationship to the closed meridian. Never expecting to discover anything so significant, I simply carried on finding the kyo stiffness of the symptom and checking which meridian it belonged to. Checking all meridian streams through my clinical practice confirmed the existence of what are now called the sub-meridians, all of which share this symmetrical relationship with what Tao Shiatsu terms the main meridians. Hence, the existence of the twenty-four meridians throughout the body was established.

The discovery of the sub-meridians also clarified the pattern of deepening kyo. Symptoms arise and first appear on the kyo main meridian. If they deepen they will appear on the sub-meridian. This solved the earlier mystery of why the symptoms had appeared on the back of the neck in the case of Large Intestine meridian kyo, rather than on the front. The sub-meridian of Large Intestine exists on the back of the neck where the patient's kyo stiffness was located.

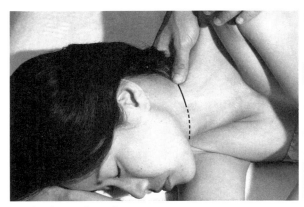

Ring kyo line on the neck.

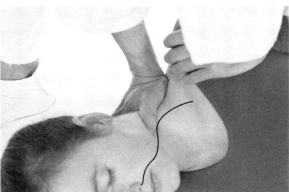

Large Intenstine meridian on the neck.

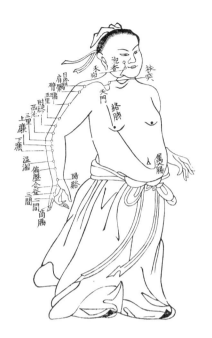

Ancient diagram of the Large Intestine meridian.

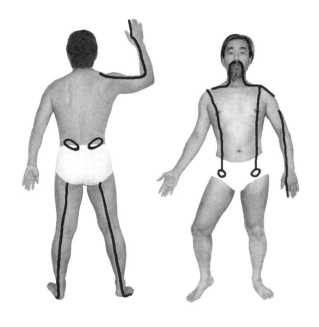

Large Intestine whole body meridian—Zen Shiatsu chart.

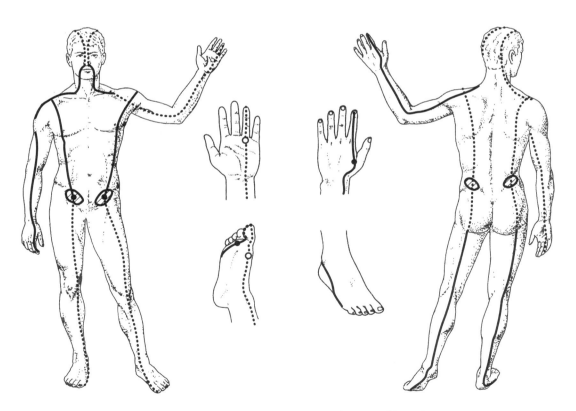

Large Intestine whole body main and sub meridian—Tao Shiatsu chart.

THE DEPTHS OF THE KI WORLD 57

Going beyond the boundaries of common sense to greater treatment effectiveness

Three years of researching tsubo in clinical practice had passed before I was able to see ki spreading and perform sho diagnosis. A further three years went by before I could see the kyo stiffness with boshin. Boshin solved the dilemma posed by the increasing number of patients in whom sho diagnosis was impossible, which was essential to giving Zen Shiatsu treatment. This covered the period around 1985 when I felt the shift in the age occurring. Another six years ensued before I could identify all twelve sub-meridians, which along with the twelve main meridians make up the twenty-four meridians for the clinical practice of Tao Shiatsu. Perhaps this seems like enough experience of the depths of the ki world for one lifetime? Yet something truly shocking was still in store for me. I was about to discover that by going deeper into the ki world, diagnosis actually became unnecessary.

A brief story that I had heard from a colleague proved to be the key that unlocked an even greater mystery, when I least expected it. He told me that on different occasions Master Masunaga had experienced a sho diagnosis revealing the Conception Vessel or Governor Vessel to be the kyo meridian. These meridians are described as extra meridians and had never been indicated as possibilities for diagnosis as the kyo meridian. The challenge to research my teacher's experience immediately arose on hearing this. When I next had a patient where the kyo meridian was difficult or impossible to diagnose, I treated the Conception Vessel. To my

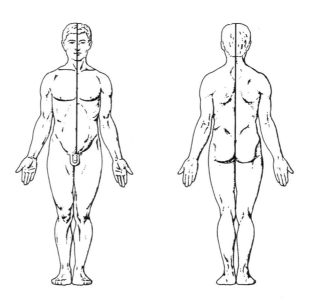

Conception Vessel and Governor Vessel lines as shown in the classical texts.

great surprise and delight the symptom was relieved; my heart was moved with gratitude for having the good fortune to have had a teacher who was a true master. However, the Conception Vessel was shown on the chart to only stream in the center of the front of the torso, which meant treatment of the hara was the only possibility. At that time many people's abdominal meridians were closed, which made their ki unresponsive to shiatsu, so in these cases I sometimes had to tell patients that they could not be treated until their kyo meridian changed.

I realized that a quantum shift in my thinking was again required, just as it had been to discover the sub-meridians. I had to release myself from the grip of the classical texts that showed the Conception Vessel to have only a center line on the front of the torso (see opposite). In clinical practice, I was treating people who displayed kyo stiffness of the Conception Vessel in both the back of the torso and in the neck. Challenging the knowledge of the classics with these clinical findings left my head spinning. For someone raised in a culture with deep reverence for the old masters and the wisdom of the classical texts, this was profoundly troubling. At the same time I have to admit it was also very exciting. Putting aside what had become "common sense" and the "conventional wisdom," I found through continued research that both the Conception and Governor Vessels also streamed in the limbs. Additionally they streamed on their opposite sides of the torso, neck, and limbs as sub-meridians (see overleaf). The meridian discoveries of Master Masunaga were being extended —the mystery of the kyo stiffness was finally resolved. Treating with this new knowledge saw treatment effectiveness immediately increase as it had with previous advances. The timing was fortuitous as it turned out, as nearly fifty percent of all my patients exhibited Conception Vessel kyo from 1989. This was in keeping with observable "trends" in the kyo meridian that seemed to change in response to the surrounding conditions.

The existence of ring and spiral meridians

A further source of confusion arose as I continued to treat the patient's symptoms through the kyo stiffness existing deep inside the kyo meridian. By now I was less surprised when kyo stiffness began to appear on lines other than the vertically flowing meridians. Frequently it now appeared on horizontal lines. The classics mention only one such meridian flowing in the hip area: this is called *taimyaku* in Japanese and constitutes another of the extra meridians. However, I was finding kyo stiffness on horizontally streaming ring meridians throughout the body. Kyo stiffness of the ring meridian did not necessarily exist along the entire line. Often only a part of the ring meridian would exhibit kyo stiffness. Having discovered a

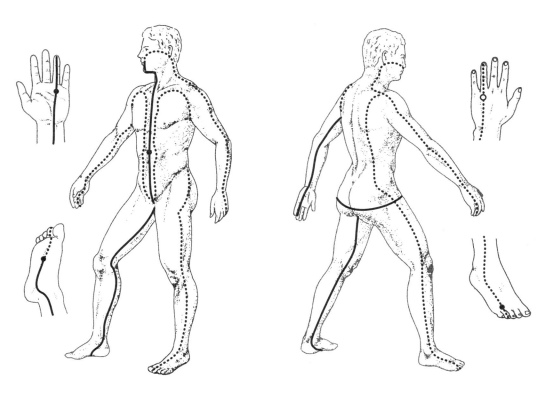

Conception Vessel—Tao Shiatsu chart showing main and sub lines.

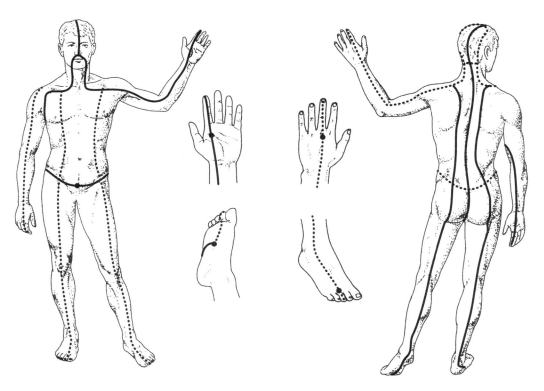

Governor Vessel—Tao Shiatsu chart showing main and sub lines.

sub-meridian for each of the main meridians led me to consider that this might also be the case for the ring meridians as well. Going ever deeper into the ki level, I found that each main meridian exhibited a series of ring meridians throughout the body. This led to further understanding of the pattern of kyo symptoms. If a symptom continues to deepen, it will go from the main meridian to the sub-meridian and then to the ring. The healing process travels in the opposite direction. Treating the kyo symptom in the ring meridian will allow it to shift to the sub-meridian. From here it will return to the main meridian where the symptom may be completely released.

The age had shifted to one in which virtually all symptoms were kyo, rather than jitsu-based. With kyo having become more and more deeply internalized, it seemed perfectly feasible that deeper meridians would be present. It is even likely that they have always existed but only now have come to our awareness out of necessity. Sub, ring, and extensions of the extra meridians—the Conception and Governor Vessels—had all revealed themselves. By this point I had grown more accepting to the appearance of meridian streams that seemed utterly beyond common sense, never mind beyond the dictates of the classics. I remembered back to the constant questioning that Master Masunaga was subjected to in the years following the publication of his chart that showed the twelve whole body meridians. Acupuncturists and Oriental medical practitioners had called him "crazy" for even suggesting such things. I could now see my own findings being subjected to similar ridicule. What I was suggesting seemed an even greater heresy in the context of the classical acupuncture meridians, where only six lines are shown in the limbs, yet even deeper meridian forms were about to present themselves. Not long afterward, I was experiencing real difficulty in finding the kyo stiffness of a patient's deepest symptom. When focusing my heart to see the patient's ki and kyo stiffness, a diagonal line began to appear. Giving shiatsu with this direction to the line relieved the kyo stiffness and revealed a *spiral* meridian stream. I had always had some sense of a spiral stream's existence from the time I was able to do boshin. It had, however, remained a subconscious feeling and never became clear, perhaps because its use in treatments was not necessary at that time. Continued research revealed that each main meridian has two spiral streams. They begin at the top of the head and end at the tip of the middle finger and the soles of the feet.

The stages of the healing process now became clear. The deepest level of the kyo symptom will appear in the spiral meridian. Treatment in this case should begin with the spiral meridian, move to the ring meridian, then the sub meridian, and finally the main meridian. The symptom transforms from kyo to jitsu and is healed. Please note that this is the theoretical process: in clinical practice people have different healing processes and exhibit variations to the theory. Being aware of this process and synchronizing it with clinical practice is what is required to see the depth of the ki world, and allow all meridian streams to become clear. At first this may seem overwhelming. However, Tao Shiatsu study and clinical treatment necessitates going beyond the horizon of common sense and limitations of the conscious mind.

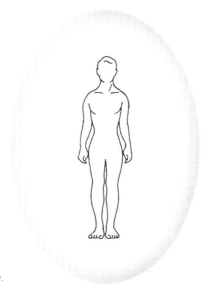

The ki body.

SIXTH STAGE
SEEING THE KI BODY

Even with the greater ease and effectiveness of shiatsu treatment, I still felt some personal resistance to these discoveries. However, it was the increased clinical effectiveness that persuaded me to present my findings. The motivation I have to teach shiatsu is simple: I hope that it is possible for people to study and practice an effective method that alleviates people's suffering. This was Master Masunaga's life work. As I continued to practice and research meridian treatment for this purpose, I finally saw the real ki depth of the meridians as being beyond the physical body: this is what Tao Shiatsu calls the "ki meridian." In fact, the Japanese kanji for Tao Shiatsu (気の経絡指圧) mean "ki meridian shiatsu."

I have always subconsciously felt that there was something deeper to ki and meridians. It has been this, coupled with Master Masunaga's work, that has driven my journey. Just as it had before, this deep sense now rose up into my consciousness with even greater clarity than when I had first seen the whole meridian. I was able to visualize the ki meridians at a depth of approximately two meters beyond the physical body, while the kyo meridian was as deep as five meters in the ki body. Subsequently I realized that the meridians we sense in the body are not in fact "meridians." They are simply the connection to the ki body—the dimension in which the meridians really exist. The kyo stiffness of the meridian we feel in our physical body is the projection of the ki meridian.

Two things concern me when discussing the ki body. One is that some people misunderstand or misinterpret the words "ki body." Others assume they understand them without any direct experience of what is being described here, or interpret them as something with New Age connotations. Secondly, as these meridians are not referred to in the classics, some see them as derived from the occult. All that I can tell you is that my clinical findings are neither manifestations of the New Age or the occult. Anyone in fact can experience the ki meridian's existence. In workshops I frequently help students give shiatsu that allows the receiver to feel the meridian depth of two meters. When ki goes through to this depth, a deep sense of comfort and feeling of something "fitting" is experienced by the receiver. Many comment that it is a sensation they have never felt through shiatsu before.

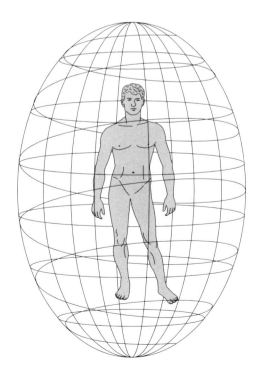

The meridian streams—vertical, ring, and spiral—exist in the ki body.

Naturally I wondered if other people had been aware of the ki body, or had written about it. During this time I came by chance across the writings of Rudolph Steiner. Steiner refers to the ethereal body, in which he described energy flowing as lines. He also wrote that blockages in these energy lines form the basis of disease. It was furthermore pointed out to me that the existence of the ki body is described in the Kabbalah of Judaism, where it is said to measure a distance of four *ammut* (about 2.24 meters) from the physical body. People have clearly been aware of the ki body since ancient times.

SEVENTH STAGE
THE EXISTENCE OF THE SUPER VESSELS

Imagine finding a different ecological life system in the depths of the ocean, something that really belonged to another dimension. This was to be my experience much deeper into the ki body. There I encountered the Super Vessels at a depth of seven meters. I felt a strange loneliness at seeing something that, as far as I knew, no one else had seen or perhaps even comprehended, including my shiatsu colleagues. I named them Super Vessels for their great importance in shiatsu treatment, and for their paradoxical nature. They are a contradiction, existing at an extreme depth, while also appearing on the periphery of the physical body where they can be recognized and confirmed by touch. Ordinarily a tsubo is physically depressed, but the tsubo on a Super Vessel are raised. There are twelve Super Vessels in total, consisting of four thick, two medium, and six thin vessels. They can be felt as ridges with varying thickness in relation to one another.

Jaki is negative energy, the ki toxins created by all life. Super Vessels protect the ki body and meridians from jaki. They further protect the giver from receiving jaki during treatment. The aim of Tao Shiatsu treatment is the energetic unification of the Super Vessel and kyo meridian in the ki body. At this depth, unification transforms jaki to seiki (vital life-supporting ki) and in some cases discharges jaki from the body. While Zen Shiatsu's meridian treatment was based on pressing the kyo meridian with empathy to discharge jaki, there was no mechanism for its conversion to seiki. Tao Shiatsu is effective in transforming jaki into seiki by using the Super Vessels in treatment.

For some time, I had also been concerned about the potential ill effects on practitioners giving shiatsu. Working with the Super Vessels significantly reduces the amount of jaki that is received by the practitioner during treatment. As a result, treatment is less tiring for the practitioner and promotes their well-being too. Furthermore, practitioners—particularly beginners—are less likely to accidentally damage the kyo meridian by pressing directly into it.

I had subconsciously been working with the Super Vessels before becoming conscious of them. In *Tao Shiatsu: Life Medicine for the 21st Century*, I described working while imagining a ki bubble so as never to press solely on the physical body. Here the move toward a conscious recognition of the Super Vessel can be glimpsed. Looking at the way Master Masunaga worked, and studying videos of his treatment, revealed that he too was subconsciously treating with the Super Vessels. Treatment effectiveness increased greatly when the subconscious understanding of the Super Vessels was unified with conscious awareness. The fatigue I had experienced from giving treatment was also significantly reduced. The Super

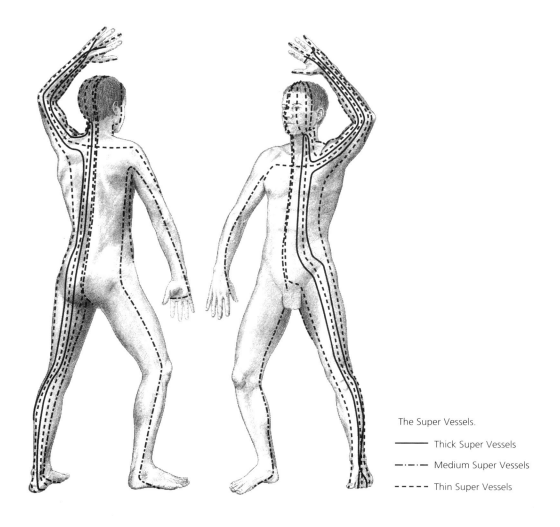

The Super Vessels.
—— Thick Super Vessels
—·—·— Medium Super Vessels
- - - - Thin Super Vessels

Vessels made me marvel at the paradox they presented: existing at such a depth, yet appearing on the body's surface where anyone could experience them. The Tao Shiatsu system and Ki Method were born with their discovery.

Jaki has various interpretations. The classics refer to its buildup as *jitsu*—ki that is stuck. All bodies create jaki and this causes the kyo–jitsu distortion of the meridian form. From this all symptoms of the mind and body arise as our bodies attempt to release jaki. Western medicine aims to control or attack these symptoms by focusing therapy directly on them through drugs, surgery, or radiation. Traditionally, Oriental medicine has aimed to balance the excessive distortion of kyo and jitsu by releasing jaki. When the giver sees deeply into their own heart the receiver's ki is revealed and so too is jaki, making it possible to direct the purpose of treatment toward changing the jaki into seiki.

Teaching about the Super Vessels is intensely challenging. At workshops, particularly in the West, participants often confront me as they struggle to "interpret" the Super Vessels. It can be most demanding for participants who are already students, practitioners, or teachers of shiatsu to accept what is being taught. People have said to me, "If I cannot grasp this in a way that makes sense, then I cannot practice what is being presented." Yet if we were to think about the computers we use, how many people can really explain what is going on inside the circuitry and software? Understanding the system is not what makes it productive or beneficial. The Super Vessels are similar. There is no need for you to logically understand them in order to work with them. If students can believe purely that they exist and then experience them directly, effective study, practice, and treatment will follow.

EIGHTH STAGE
JAKI AND ITS ESSENCE

I only sensed the Super Vessels (not consciously recognized) now and again prior to my heart state deepening at the second stage. With jaki it was very different. I felt its presence clearly all around. Habitual ki—or karma, as Buddhism might describe jaki—accumulates from the cause-and-effect nature of life. A fundamental Buddhist belief is that to be born a human is to inherit the karma of all humanity. This energy carries over from previous lives and includes ancestral karma. As this aspect is not directly necessary for giving shiatsu treatment, I had never investigated it further.

Jaki is energy from the source of existence. In seeking to release this energy, the kyo–jitsu distortion in the meridians is created. A still deeper and more direct recognition of my heart and the ki world now showed me where jaki existed in the body, and how it affected the meridians. The way to locate and treat jaki is through special points named Super Vessel Specific Tsubo ("SST"). Patients feel the strongest echoes and greatest release of pain and kyo stiffness when the SST are treated. For Tao Shiatsu study and practice, eighteen areas of the body have been identified that contain this special form of tsubo, and these are outlined in chapter six. Starting to treat jaki using the SST made me feel that it was no longer necessary to diagnose the kyo meridian to give effective treatment.

I wondered if this discovery, which brought me face-to-face with the reality of jaki, was the end of the journey. Could it be that this is really the final state of the ki world? If the ki body extended out two meters from the physical body, while the Super Vessels are at such a deep level that they can be recognized on the body's surface, what was the depth of jaki? It also existed at a very deep level while being present inside the physical body too. If the deepest level of the ki world was jaki, then the essence of ki is karma. To reach a conclusion that jaki is the source of all existence seemed very sad—thankfully, that was not the case. What was finally revealed is deeper than the ki world itself: the existence of what I, as a Buddhist, recognize as Buddha-nature. This universal, all-pervasive, and infinite spiritual energy is the essence of jaki. While jaki is experienced in the body as dysfunctional and disruptive to daily health, from inside the deepest level of the ki world it is beyond positive or negative. By investigating only within the ki world, I had placed a limitation on seeing and grasping the essence of jaki. It is beyond the ki world. The development of Tao Shiatsu was guided by my spiritual training, through the Buddhist meditation practice of *nembutsu* chanting, and it was this that revealed the essence of jaki for me. The final state of the ki world is the Buddha-nature—or Christ-heart, the equivalent concept in an alternative religious tradition, such as Christianity.

Reading another person's heart

Around the time I began to study shiatsu I commenced Buddhist practice. While researching the ki world through shiatsu, I continued to train in the Jodo (Pure Land) tradition of Buddhism. In 1991, following completion of the formal training, I became a Jodo priest. The depth and infinite nature of the state of enlightenment were glimpsed through this training, as was the state and direction of the heart needed to perceive it. A great temptation is aroused when the primal sense is awakened. Seeing ki and performing sho diagnosis can be easily mistaken as a state of enlightenment, just as easily as it is to fall into the trap of believing that some degree of self-ability is involved. I feel very fortunate that this did not happen to me during these experiences and discoveries. Buddhism describes the capacity to see ki, read auras, experience past lives, or foretell the future, as aspects of the Heavenly State—but this is not an enlightened state. It remains linked to the world of samsara—the cycle of karma still governed by the law of cause and effect. To misinterpret as enlightenment what might be perceived as "super-natural" powers, leads to much harm and increased suffering. Even the sutras, which contain the writings central to Buddhism, warn that people are still bound by karma and samsara when the primal sense is awakened. Guruism arises when a teacher uses the demonstration of special powers or miracles to convince others of their "unique ability." People are stimulated to follow the teacher in order to discover this ability. However, the enlightened state of Buddhahood is a level beyond the Heavenly State: it is where desire is overcome and the mind relieved from all attachment.

It is the primal sense that is awakened at the third stage of boshin, when moment-to-moment changes in another person's heart can be seen. During teaching and treatment, I am able to see the student and patient's heart state and the changing pattern of ki. Suggestions then arise from my subconscious that can help and guide people's study and healing. Being able to point out to people what is in their subconscious helps them to see it as well. The student's empathetic imagination toward their teacher (and other students) deepens as a result, enabling more direct transmission of the teachings. In shiatsu treatment the receiver, through deepening ki unification with the giver, is able to realize more clearly the source of their pain or disease.

Beyond physical form, technique, and conscious knowledge, is the form of the heart. This is the ki and spirit of the tradition that is transmitted in a continuous stream from generation to generation. Tao Shiatsu teaching and training is based on this transmission of ki from teacher to student. Seeing the student's ki allows the teacher to help the student to receive the tradition, which they had in turn received from their teacher. The capacity to fully appreciate and receive the teachings grows in this way, leading to the increased effectiveness of the Ki Method. Although this sounds like an ideal process, it is not always so. People in seminars and classes often have very strong egos and assert themselves and their opinions forcefully. Whether consciously or subconsciously, it creates a lot of negativity and is very tiring. I most certainly am not enlightened. It is only when teaching or giving treatment that I am able to see ki. In daily life I am as vulnerable as the next person to getting lost in new cities when I travel. I sometimes wish that when abroad I was afforded some special protection against losing my way or being cheated by taxi drivers. Unfortunately this is not the case. So I live in hope that one day this way of seeing might extend to my everyday life.

The ki world and its depths are revealed through the unity of subject and object, giver and receiver. Seeing and feeling what you do not see and feel in daily life results from going deeper into this world. Awakening the primal sense is the starting point for seeing ki. This leads toward the universal state of Buddha-nature.

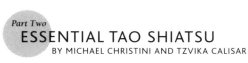

Part Two
ESSENTIAL TAO SHIATSU
BY MICHAEL CHRISTINI AND TZVIKA CALISAR

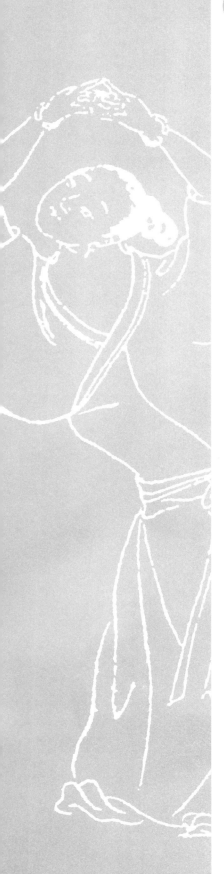

4

THE HEART OF TAO

THE FIVE ELEMENTS OF TAO SHIATSU

The heart of *sesshin* as taught by Master Masunaga and other past masters is the source of Tao Shiatsu. The study and practice of Tao Shiatsu consists of Five Elements, each with a method and principles to follow. These Five Elements are: 1) Ki Doin, 2) tsubo and SST treatment, 3) Super Vessel recognition and Ki Method treatment, 4) kyo meridian treatment, and 5) Basic Forms, and they will be discussed in the following chapters. While all the Ki Methods have practical steps to adhere to, if they are used as instruction manuals they will not work. The effectiveness of Tao Shiatsu depends on the practitioner receiving and developing the heart of Tao. The universal qualities of this heart are faith, gratitude, generosity, devotion, and humility. Healing does not arise from technical proficiency, and understanding this is the key to successful study and practice. All of the traditional Eastern disciplines—from the tea ceremony to meditation and martial artistry—share one common purpose: the spiritual development of the practitioner through repeated practice and refinement of form and technique, in order that this may benefit the spiritual development of others. Practice of these arts strengthens and deepens the Tao heart that we all possess, and allows the oneness of heart and body to be realized. Once this occurs, the aim of Tao Shiatsu treatment—to unify the patient's heart and body—becomes possible. Shiatsu where the focus of study is on acquiring technique and knowledge will never be fully effective, no matter how much time and effort is applied to it. Developing the Tao heart is what allows meridian recognition and effective treatment to take place. The teachings of Tao Shiatsu are primarily concerned with the transmission of the spirit of sesshin and the heart of Tao, rather than simply technique alone. In all honesty, cultivating this heart requires time, perseverance, and devotion.

THE HEART OF SESSHIN

Sesshin is the most essential aspect of Oriental diagnosis and what distinguishes it from other forms, yet even practitioners of Oriental medicine frequently misunderstand its true essence. When Master Masunaga reflected on the development of shiatsu as a therapy, he felt it necessary to point out that sesshin, especially in terms of common acupuncture practice, had come to mean little more than "touch" diagnosis. This is "touch" in the same sense as the manual examination carried out in Western medicine. This is far removed from the meaning of sesshin—while there may be parallels at a superficial level, the approach is actually completely different. To understand this difference, it is very revealing to look at the kanji for *shokushin*, the Japanese term for Western medical touch diagnosis. One of the elements making up the character represents an insect's antenna, as mentioned earlier. Its purpose is to identify external threats toward its owner, which parallels the role of the sense of touch in Western medical diagnosis: the search for any discernable abnormality.

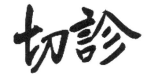

The kanji for *sesshin*.

Like shokushin, performing sesshin also requires direct contact with the patient's body, often pressing with the hands and fingers, as in shiatsu. Here, however, the similarity ends: sesshin is performed in an entirely different heart state. It seeks to understand the situation of the meridians empathetically—by feeling the other person's life sensation as if it were your own. The physical sense of touch is based on the conscious ego and sesshin can never be performed through it. In Western medicine, judging what is normal or abnormal in the patient's condition is performed in a state of separation between practitioner and patient. The very nature of objective examination is for the observer to be independent of what is observed. A fundamentally different approach is needed for sesshin: it is necessary to be of one heart and mind with the receiver so as to empathetically imagine what they are feeling, and to really want to deeply understand and share the other person's life. Awakening the primal sense is absolutely essential for the practitioner to clearly see the receiver's meridian state.

Sesshin's original meaning in Japanese is "to cut." One element making up the kanji represents a knife. In the context of diagnosis, this represents the wish to share another person's life so deeply that it is "cutting to the core of one's heart." An egoless heart state creates a level of empathy that reaches such a depth that the ki bodies become one. Even though there is physical contact, any sense of a border between the giver and receiver disappears. Importantly, the giver does not consciously recognize how deep their empathy is. There is no sense of self-ability when the bottom of the tsubo and meridian are revealed.

THE FIVE-THOUSAND-YEAR-OLD STREAM OF ORIENTAL MEDICINE

The heart of Tao can only be developed through meaningful study and practice leading to the direct realization that this heart is dwelling deep inside each and every being. The actual feeling of the Tao heart must be experienced. Modern shiatsu has received the gift of the spirit and the heart of sesshin diagnosis from Master Masunaga. Whoever truly receives this heart and spirit will not think of it as a product of their own ability. If there is even a mere hint of doubt about this, it is clearly not the spirit transmitted through the master. Internally awakening this heart opens the gateway to a vast unceasing stream. The actual feeling experienced by the master who received this stream is, in turn, experienced by their student. Transmission may occur without having actually met the master directly, as is evident in the Mahayana Buddhist sutras, which almost invariably begin with the words, "I heard this from Buddha." Even sutras recorded many hundreds of years after the Buddha's death, and clearly not the actual spoken words of Gautama Buddha, contain this. The writers of the sutras convey the realization that the wisdom of enlightenment contained in them was received from the heart of Buddha. When I received the capacity to perform sho diagnosis, I experienced the actual feeling of Master Masunaga's heart state even though he had passed away by that time. Direct contact with the teacher is not an absolute requirement. Transmission may occur through the words and images of a book that express the master's teachings. A relationship between master and student exists when there is appreciation and absolute realization of the means by which the heart of Tao is received. Whether or not a student is able to perform sho diagnosis, effective treatment with Tao Shiatsu becomes possible with wholehearted faith in Tao and adherence to the method.

For over twenty years I have tried to work in this way, treating patients one by one while researching and teaching. At times there were only a handful of students in my classes, yet I continued to investigate the method and adapted it in order to find the clearest transmission. Of course, not all students continued studying. Many gave up or lost interest. Only a few of my early students grew into the roles of practitioner and teacher. Yet now, as Tao Shiatsu spreads throughout the world, the heart of Tao and the real spirit of Oriental medicine are being received by more students for healing and transmission to others.

RECEIVE TAO KI DIRECTLY INTO YOUR HEART

Certified instructors teach Tao Shiatsu at centers around the world. All classes follow common principles and methods, allowing students to study anywhere and receive the same teachings. The only real obstacle to study, then, is whether the student is determined to confront their heart and follow the way of Tao. For example, students find they are able to locate tsubo or Super Vessels and give treatment when they first begin attending classes. On returning home and practicing on friends and family, however, they discover, to their confusion, and sometimes frustration, that they are unable to repeat this experience. Why could the receiver in the classroom feel the tsubo and ki reaching the bottom, but now this is difficult or impossible to achieve? Everyone faces this dilemma and must consider what is happening. Therein lies the key to being a student. Ordinarily common sense would tell you that the method should work if you attend class, study it, and continue to practice. If this is not the case, a common response is to blame the method, or to feel that "you" are not good enough to do it. Both interpretations miss what is really happening. Students receive ki directly to their subconscious through the teacher, who in turn has received this ki from their teacher. This is the ki of Tao. Tao Shiatsu teachers try to allow Tao ki to penetrate the subconscious of everyone in the class, and students are able to do the method for this reason. Tao heart and spirit are present. This is the unbroken stream of ki flowing through five thousand years of Oriental medical practice, transmitted from teacher to student through the ages. As long as the heart is open, the transmission of ki enables students to do the method. The methods introduced in this book may appear to be set out as manuals, but it is a real mistake to use them in this way. While effective meridian treatment becomes possible by following the steps of the method in class, it has nothing to do with the student's ability. In the class there is a teacher and the ki of Tao is present. The methods of Tao Shiatsu exist and work only with the ki and heart of Tao. If you practice only with the words, forms, and techniques, Tao Shiatsu does not happen. Ki will not reach the bottom of the receiver's kyo meridian. This is what distinguishes Tao Shiatsu from the previous forms of physically therapeutic shiatsu and why the Tao Shiatsu methods that will be explained in the following chapters are called the Ki Method. Teaching Tao Shiatsu comes from mastering the way of receiving ki from Tao so that others may also receive it.

THE POWER OF IMAGINATION IS THE WAY TO RECEIVE THE KI METHOD

Your imagination can be the basis of a method that allows you to receive the ki of Tao through the images in this book. To achieve this, you must study the photographs illustrating the methods with more than just your eyes and consciousness: in addition to looking at the physical form of each picture, try to imagine the ki and heart state of the teacher at all times. This allows ki from the Tao to penetrate to your subconscious.

What function of ki creates the mechanism that makes this possible? First, consider the way in which people in Japan customarily entered into the study of the arts. Traditionally, training ki is a necessary component of all art forms, be it calligraphy, poetry, painting, the tea ceremony, or a martial art. Initially the teacher or master may have given almost no formal instruction to the student. The student lived in the master's house or school and went about daily life activities while observing how the master was working. Simply by spending their time around the master, carefully observing and attending to the form and detail of the master's actions, the student received ki through words and images directly into their subconscious. When these images started to rise to the surface, they were expressed in the ki and actions of the student, who was eventually able to work in the same or a similar way as the master.

On a more mundane level, this process is illustrated by the behavior that moviegoers frequently exhibit after seeing a movie. An example often seen in Japan, following the screening of a *yakuza* (mafia) movie, is the rolling movement of the shoulders and exaggerated position of the jaw displayed by some of the men leaving the theater. Just think of a movie that has really affected or moved you and I am sure everyone will have had a similar experience at one time or another. The ki of a character "enters" into your subconscious and you find yourself trying to mimic their speech or movement. In my own case I have to admit that one of my favorite films is *Being There*, starring Peter Sellers. When it first came out, I saw it five times in one day! One week later, I was still copying the character's funny way of talking and still find myself doing it sometimes, even now! While such an example may seem a little trivial, it clearly illustrates the point that ki can be received through an image.

A further example of this mechanism is the image training of Mahayana Buddhism. Continuously imagining the form of Buddha during meditation leads to the awakening of the universal spirit of Buddha nature and its expansion in the heart.

Try working with this method of image training by using the photos in the book. Look at each picture and activate the subconscious by trying to

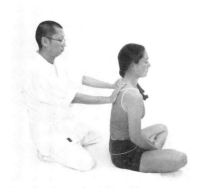

Imagine the teacher's ki and heart state, not just the physical form.

imagine the teacher's ki and heart state. Practicing the method this way will allow the teacher's ki to penetrate your heart. Imagining this constantly while practicing will begin to influence your subconscious.

Two aspects are vital to keep in mind:

1. The influence of ki is always much more than we think, so avoid being too quick to underestimate the effect of this practice.
2. Ki always follows the image. Therefore try to form the image as clearly and deeply as possible.

Tao Shiatsu has three levels of practitioner training. The methods and images of this book are, for the most part, concerned with the entrance level of Tao Shiatsu. However, even the entrance level can include the advanced level. It all depends on the student's attitude.

Tao Shiatsu's methods work only by receiving the ki of Tao: this is the way to receive mastery of Tao Shiatsu. Without this realization, there is only the dependence on self-ability and personal capacity, which will create a situation where in one moment it is able to be done, and then it disappears.

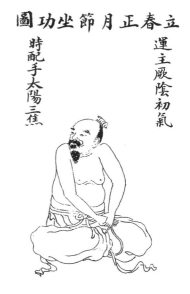

FIRST ELEMENT
Ki Doin
—Increase the Power and Potential of Ki

Ki Doin is the first of Tao Shiatsu's Five Elements studied at the entrance level. Its origins, and those of shiatsu, lie in the ancient system of Doin Ankyo. In China, the tradition had existed where specialist practitioners of energy cultivation (*doin*), who resided in the mountains where they developed these skills, would come down into the cities and give medical treatment (*ankyo*). Doin was comprised of three broad disciplines: ki exercise forms resembling yoga and qigong, martial artistry, and the practice of meditation. Ankyo consisted of the practices of *anma* (massage) and *kyosei* (physical manipulation). Shiatsu's original form was the hand pressure method that developed from anma and incorporated the practice of kyosei. Over time the practice of Doin Ankyo in its original form almost completely disappeared. Recently, however, increasing numbers of schools of Oriental medicine in China have reintroduced qigong and doin as compulsory core subjects in their curriculum. This points the way to a revival of these practices as a central part of Oriental medicine.

Enriching our own ki is the way to develop the capacity to assist others to strengthen their ki. This is obviously one significant reason for doin's value to the practice of shiatsu. Additionally, Ki Doin's great importance to

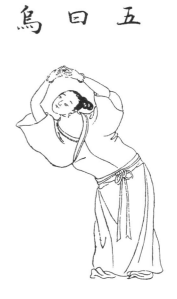

Ancient *doin* diagrams.

Tao Shiatsu is that it forms a direct way for students to study the principles of the Ki Method of shiatsu. The principles of Ki Doin form the basis of the Ki Method, supporting and reinforcing it. Patients receiving treatment are also able to practice Ki Doin to assist their recovery and healing.

Ki Doin consists of four main aspects: Renki, Aiki, Meridian Yoga, and Ki Breathing meditation. Renki has seven individual ki movement exercises, and is performed at two different speeds: the yin practice is very slow, like Tai Chi, and the yang practice much faster. Aiki, which has seven forms, is based on martial arts practices and is performed with a partner. Meridian Yoga is a series of energetic partner-assisted stretches for the meridians. Ki Breathing is a meditation practice.

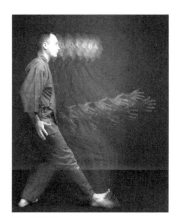

The Ki Ball.

THE PRINCIPLES OF RENKI

There are important principles governing the exchange of human ki and the way it can be purified and enriched.

FIRST KI PRINCIPLE
SYNCHRONIZATION

Synchronization involves maintaining the oneness of the body's external movement with the internal image. Practically, this requires the practitioner to make the physical movement of the arms and lower body the same speed. Concentrating the mind on the image of each principle while unifying it with the physical sensation develops the unity of heart and body. As this

RENKI PRACTICE: THE KI BALL.

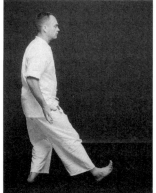 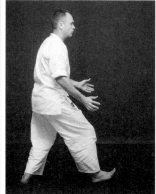 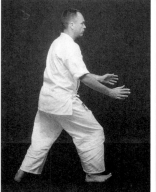 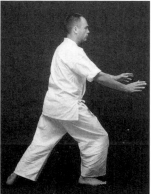

1. Stand with your right foot forward and the toe up. Imagine holding a ball of ki.

2. Begin to move the ball forward. The hands turn around the center fingers, with movement synchronized with the toe coming down toward the ground.

3. Keep pushing the ball forward and parallel to the ground.

4. Arms are extended and stop moving forward at the same time the toe touches the ground. The left heel remains on the ground throughout. Keep holding the ball while reversing the movement to return to the starting position.

sense of unity evolves, the practitioner begins to feel the sense of the ki body extending outward in all directions from the physical body.

Practice with the Ki Ball and synchronization principle. Physically, the hands move forward turning around the middle finger at the same speed as the front foot comes down to the floor. Then reverse.

Hakkiho: experimenting with the strength of ki

Hakkiho is a method for testing and experimenting with the strength of ki that is channeled as the practitioner works with the ki principles. Find a willing partner and let us begin with the Ki Ball exercise and the principle of synchronization.

Hakkiho with the Ki Ball

1. Giver stands behind the receiver in a relaxed manner. Imagine yourself as a tree. Drop your point of awareness (ki center) while keeping your torso straight and upright.

2. Place your hands on the back of your partner.

3. First push using your physical strength and see how far your partner moves.

4. Now synchronize the movement of your arms with your lower body, while imagining the strength flowing from your lower body (rather than from your arms), to move the receiver.

RENKI PRACTICE: HAKKIHO WITH THE KI BALL.

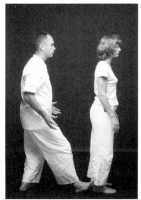 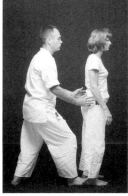 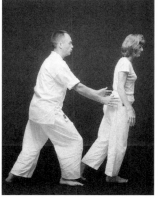 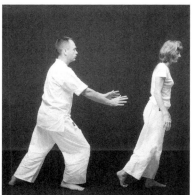

If performed correctly the receiver moves much further, and feels more comfortable, when the ki principle is used to perform the movement. Please note that it is very important that the receiver is not stubborn. Rather than

RENKI PRACTICE: INFINITY EIGHT.

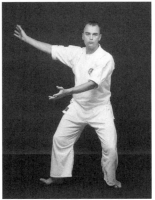 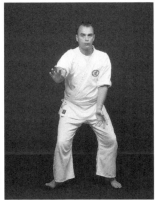 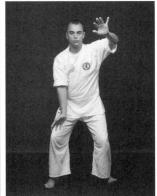 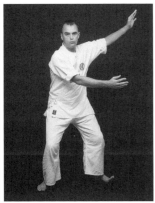

1. Stand with your feet shoulder-width apart and right toes up. Bring your right arm up and left arm lower down.

2. Move your arms downward, turning around the center fingers, as though moving around a pipe looped in a figure eight.

3. Move through the center of the eight to the lowest point. Come up on the other side, with the left arm leading, left foot coming up.

4. The left arm and left foot are now up. Reverse the movement completing the figure eight by returning to the start position.

RENKI PRACTICE: THE SUNFLOWER.

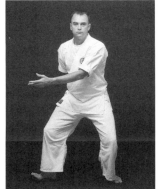 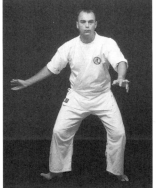 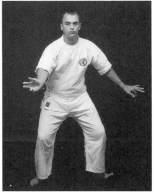 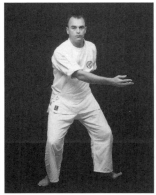

1. Stand with feet shoulder-width apart. Bend your knees and drop your center of gravity. Right toe is up, with left arm across the body, right arm behind.

2. Turn through your center line with movement coming from the seika tanden, and let your arms follow.

3. Right toe comes down and left toe starts to come up.

4. Right arm is now across the body and left toe is now up. Reverse movement and return to starting position.

RENKI PRACTICE: THE WATERFALL.

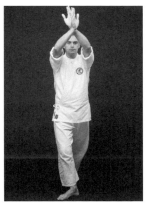 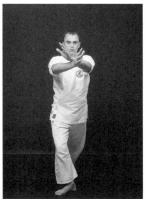 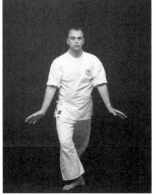 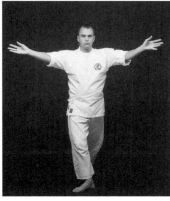

1. Step forward with your right foot and turn feet slightly outward. Raise your back heel up off the ground, so the front leg straightens. Bring your hands up above your head with the wrists crossed.

2. The hands come down, crossing in front of the chest, and are synchronized with the back heel coming down toward the floor.

3. As the hands reach the bottom of the movement, your heel touches the floor. The front leg is now bent. The back leg always remains straight.

4. The hands now move upward with the same speed as the heel coming up. Return to the start position.

resisting the efforts of the giver, try to follow and adapt to their ki. Resisting is not good for the well-being of either the giver or the receiver. All the principles can be practiced with hakkiho. The increasing strength of ki can be experienced as each new principle is added during practice. All seven Renki exercises have hakkiho forms.

As each of the following ki principles is introduced, practice it with the Ki Ball. Add the new principle to the preceding principles so that the effect is cumulative.

SECOND KI PRINCIPLE
CONTROLLING THE MOVEMENT OF THE TANDEN

The *tanden* are the major energy centers where the body internally creates the life-giving energy that maintains health. The kanji depicting tanden (丹田) can be translated as "medicine field/farm."

The *seika*—or lower—tanden is located just below the navel, inside the center of the torso in front of the spine. The upper tanden is located inside the forehead and is often referred to as the third eye. The middle tanden is known as *danchu* and is located inside the center of the chest between the nipples.

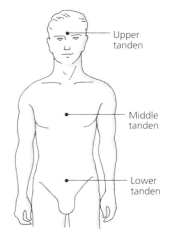

In addition to these three major tanden, Tao Shiatsu has also identified the bottom tanden. This point exists at the very bottom of the ki body, approximately two meters below the lowest point of the physical body. In the Renki exercises, it is the movement of the seika tanden that is focused on. Controlling its movement is vitally important for training ki. In Tai Chi training, for example, the aim is to move the tanden parallel to the ground, but in Renki four directions of tanden movement are practiced:

1. Parallel to the ground for the Ki Ball and Spiral Punch.

2. Perpendicular to the ground for the Waterfall.

3. Rotating at the same location for the Sunflower, Dynamic Spin, and Cross Cut.

4. Turning in the pattern of Infinity Eight.

NOTE: Spiral Punch, Dynamic Spin, and Cross Cut are not pictured. Visit www.taoshiatsu.com to view these exercises.

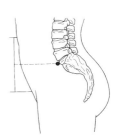

Seika tanden.

Now practice hakkiho for the Ki Ball, and with image and action move the seika tanden parallel to the ground.

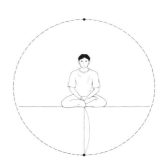

Bottom tanden.

THE HEART OF TAO 79

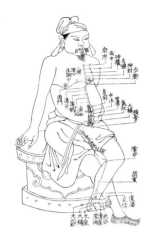

Ancient diagram of the Kidney meridian.

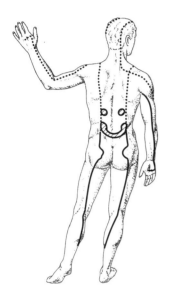

The Kidney meridian: Tao Shiatsu chart.

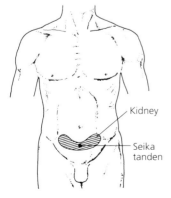

Hara diagram of the Kidney meridian area and seika tanden.

THIRD KI PRINCIPLE
USING THE KIDNEY MERIDIAN TO STRENGTHEN KI

Emphasizing only one of the twelve meridians and giving it its own principle may seem unusual. However, in *The Yellow Emperor*—Oriental medicine's most famous classical text—it is written that the universal ki of nature first enters the meridian system through the Kidney meridian. Furthermore, the energy of the Kidney meridian governs the aging process, weakening as we grow older and disappearing when we die. It is related to the functioning of the hormonal system, the hair, bones, teeth, eyesight, sexual vitality, and fertility. Taoism's philosophy and practice of promoting longevity strongly emphasizes that the tanden be exercised to slow down the aging process. There are numerous examples of Taoist practitioners in Taiwan who at the age of eighty still look only half their age. To achieve such feats, controlling and reducing stress is emphasized, as it is very detrimental to the Kidney energy. So too are coffee and white sugar, which are considered toxic to healthy Kidney energy. The following charts show the pathway of the Kidney meridian as depicted by the classical and Tao meridian charts.

Note that the Classical meridian chart depicts the Kidney meridian flowing only in the legs, while the Tao Shiatsu meridian chart shows it flowing in the arms as well. This resulted from Master Masunaga's discovery that all twelve meridian channels existed throughout the body. It was further confirmed for me when I realized that the traditional form of kyudo archery also utilized the Kidney line in the arm. Archers have never formally described it as relating to the arm Kidney line, but they connect to it through the highly refined distinguishing sense that they possess as martial artists.

The Tao Shiatsu hara chart shows the central diagnosis point of each meridian. Looking carefully at this reveals that the Kidney meridian point passes through the same location as the seika tanden. In the previous principle it was seen that the seika tanden is the center for all movement of the body. The fact that the meridian exists as an aspect of the ki world, where no distance exists, makes this principle possible. Real ki strength is developed by imagining the arm Kidney line synchronized with the leg Kidney line and with the seika tanden as the center of movement. To perform this principle, at the beginning of movement concentrate on the arm Kidney line, then from the turning point shift awareness to the leg Kidney line. This same principle is working in the Ki Method for shiatsu when taking the Super Vessel to the bottom of kyo. Practice shifting awareness from arm Kidney to leg Kidney with the Ki Ball.

FOURTH KI PRINCIPLE
INCREASE SPEED

Ki is not physical matter and exists only in the state of constant motion, as was famously expressed by Albert Einstein's equation $E=mc^2$. Existence is itself only happening through ki. Discoveries in quantum physics are confirming what has long been held to be true by Eastern philosophy. Everything in the whole universe is in a state of unceasing movement: nothing remains still. If ki exists only in a state of motion, then there must be a speed at which it moves fastest. Rather than looking at this purely as a mathematical measurement, in terms of distance per second, what is the form of speed that most extends ki? What might be called pendulum speed is the most natural speed and is common to all of existence. This is the speed created by the force of gravity, which increases naturally at the rate of thirty-two feet per second on earth and was discovered by the physicist Bloom. However, in the practice of the Renki exercises there is no need for exact numbers. Just keep imagining the speed increasing with the speed of a pendulum. In daily life this natural increase in speed can be witnessed when objects are dropped and fall under gravity. In the sweeping motion of a broom, when it is performed unconsciously, the stroke of the broom naturally increases speed. Shinto priests in Japan can be seen performing purification rituals to clean up the ki of places or objects. They do this by means of strings of paper attached to sticks, which they wave back and forth with increasing speed. In Renki, the turning point from arm to leg of the Kidney principle is the point at which speed begins to increase.

In the Ki Method, from the point of touching the surface to reaching the bottom of tsubo, the time is only a couple of seconds and the physical distance that the thumb moves is only from a half to one centimeter: however, the arm Kidney shifts to the leg Kidney with increasing speed. It can be clearly seen that principles of Renki (*doin*) are deeply connected to the Ki Method (*ankyo*), with movement the same in both cases. It creates the oneness with yin (Renki) and yang (Ki Method).

- Practice increasing speed from the turning point with the Ki Ball.
- Practice the other three Renki exercises shown with all four ki principles.

For daily Renki practice, six revolutions of the movement are practiced with each principle in those exercises where there is no need to change sides, such as Sunflower and Infinity Eight. Three revolutions of the movement are practiced for the other exercises where all principles are practiced first on the right side and then on the left, such as with Ki Ball and Waterfall.

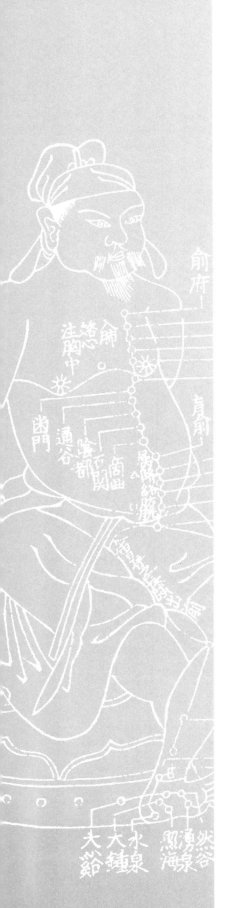

5

ESSENTIALS OF TREATMENT

SECOND ELEMENT
The Tsubo Method

Tsubo treatment is the second of the Five Elements studied at the entrance level of Tao Shiatsu. Unification of heart, image, and action is the basis of all training. Giving effective treatment is not about studying the meridian chart to learn the position of tsubo to press. While this perception and practice is common, real meridian treatment through tsubo is an entirely different process of developing the heart state to actually see the meridians.

THE TSUBO METHOD FOR EFFECTIVE MERIDIAN TREATMENT

Tao Shiatsu training makes it possible, even at the entrance level of study, to give meridian treatment without any prior knowledge of the names, functions, or imbalances of the meridians. Just one heart is needed to find tsubo: the heart that can deeply imagine where the receiver most wants to be pressed. Just one heart is needed to press the tsubo: the heart that can continuously imagine how the receiver is feeling each moment. The focus of study is to eliminate any gap between the three dimensions of human life: the heart state, the image, and the physical action. Essentially, though, the heart is the base and determines the depth of healing that results for the receiver.

For many people it is a new experience to deeply imagine how someone else is feeling at each moment while maintaining physical contact. In Tao Shiatsu it is called empathetic imagination. It becomes weaker when not experienced regularly, or when people are unable or unwilling to feel the pain of others due to selfishness. To practice empathetic imagination you must try to look clearly at your heart and see it each moment, while at the same time trying to imagine what the receiver is feeling subconsciously. Shiatsu is much more than just applying physical pressure to points on the body. Empathetic imagination is what the meridian responds to, and what makes meridian treatment with shiatsu effective.

THE WAY TO FIND KI TSUBO

Tsubo are the gateway to meridian shiatsu and can be found by anyone through empathetic imagination. Feedback received from people after the first Tao Shiatsu book was published in 1995 revealed that many people were still unable to find the tsubo that were described. In most cases, it appeared that tsubo were still being approached as though they were something to be located in the physical body. Given society's emphasis on the physical existence of the material body, this is quite understandable.

Before starting practice, clearly understand that each tsubo includes the whole of the physical and ki bodies. The real depth of the tsubo is the ki tsubo: it exists simultaneously at the outer border of the receiver's ki body, and at a corresponding depth in the subconscious of both giver and receiver. Using the middle finger, rather than the index finger or thumb, allows the giver's ki to most clearly reach the tsubo's real depth.

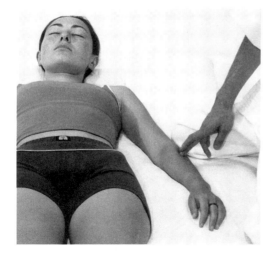

LOCATING KI TSUBO

1. Look at the area shown in the lower arm.
2. Imagine the place where the receiver most wants to be pressed.
3. Use the middle finger to touch and confirm the ki tsubo.

If you experienced difficulty in this exercise, consider where it comes from. Doubt or inability to comprehend ki tsubo will obviously make experiencing them impossible. If people are unwilling to look into their heart—to see what intention, feeling, or motivation is being expressed by it—the ki world will remain closed. If there is any thought that the tsubo can be found with self-ability, the exercise will also be difficult. As described earlier, students often experience the ki tsubo clearly in classes and seminars, but find they are unable to do so outside of the class. The heart that allows the tsubo to be felt cannot be created, no matter how much you try. It comes from the Tao and is received only by the transmission from teacher to student.

While it is clearly not possible for everyone reading this book to attend a class with a teacher at this moment, the opportunity still exists to study in the way described. As outlined earlier, the process is available to anyone through the images contained in the following photos, which can make it possible for you to receive the heart to locate and feel tsubo. First, though, you must realize how much we are influenced by the illusion that the body is matter and that our consciousness determines the reality we experience. The power of the ego, and our overreliance on it, leads to the perception that all action is a matter of individual ability. When ego becomes the center of human existence, separation from the heart occurs. This leads to separation of the self from others.

THE STEPS IN TSUBO TREATMENT

The illustrations show the instructor demonstrating the steps involved in locating tsubo. Look at each photo and try to imagine the heart and action that the teacher is working with. Then practice the steps in the same way.

LOCATING TSUBO THROUGH THE IMAGE OF THE TEACHER

1. Imagine the place where the receiver most wants to be pressed.
2. Touch with the middle finger while imagining how the receiver feels. The degree of pressure—in the physical sense—should reach somewhere between the depth of the skin and muscle. Let empathetic imagination determine this depth.
3. Move the finger slightly back and forth and sideways, while imagining how the receiver is feeling. Ask the receiver if they feel the tsubo responding and try to feel the rice tip.

Please remember, the tsubo belongs to the meridian—the ki pathway: it is not physical matter. The tsubo never responds if approached or pressed only as a physical dimension.

A mixture of doubt and belief is a frequent response of people when they see or experience the real nature of tsubo and how it is revealed to the giver's heart through empathetic imagination. They reply with a hesitant "uh-huh" rather than a definite "yes" when asked about it. Even after directly experiencing the clear difference between physical pressure and empathetic imagination, people's hearts do not change immediately. Some people are initially impressed by the experience, but quickly return to the habit of pressing physically. Others doubt and wonder if the experience is real or not, even after the receiver has assured them that it was completely different when location and treatment were performed with empathetic imagination.

Tsubo have been described as "a knot in a piece of string," or "the tip of a rice grain." Just accept the way it feels to you, and avoid interpreting or rationalizing it, such as deciding that what you are feeling must be muscle. Then again, steer clear of the opposite extreme of thinking it must be something very special or mystical. Just do not "think too much" about it!

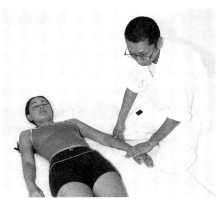

Step 2 (i): Find the best angle—touch the tsubo with the thumb and allow the elbows to naturally bend by moving toward the receiver.

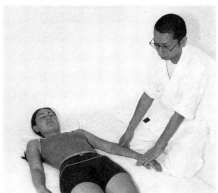

Step 2 (ii): Find the best angle—keep touching the tsubo with the thumb. Move with empathetic imagination back from the receiver until you naturally stop. This is the best angle.

TREATING TSUBO WITH THE TSUBO METHOD

1. Locate and touch the tsubo with your middle finger. Confirm the tsubo is open.
    - A tsubo that is open will echo when it is pressed (see p. 33). If the receiver feels no echo, then the tsubo cannot be treated.
    - Being able to imagine the receiver's whole body through the tsubo also indicates that the tsubo is open and effective treatment is possible. When only a part of the body can be imagined, then the tsubo is closed.
2. Find the best angle of the elbow to allow ki to go through.
    - Touch the tsubo with your thumb and support the receiver's body with the other hand.
    - Keep touching the tsubo, relax your upper body, and move it toward the receiver so that your elbows bend.
    - Find the best angle of the elbow by moving slowly back from the receiver with empathetic imagination until your body naturally stops moving. This is the best angle to allow ki to reach the bottom of the tsubo.

3. Locate the tsubo that exists inside the tsubo.
   - Lift your thumb off the tsubo briefly without any fear of losing it.
   - Locate the tsubo again by imagining where the receiver most wants to be pressed *inside* the tsubo you had been touching.
   - Touch this tsubo, which exists within the first tsubo, with your thumb.
   - The sensation of the tsubo should now be much clearer for the receiver.
4. Allow ki to reach the bottom of the tsubo.
   - Keep imagining how the receiver is feeling each moment and press, by straightening your elbow, to allow ki to reach the bottom of the tsubo.
5. Adapt to release jaki when the sensation of ki pressing back against your thumb is felt.

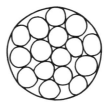

Step 3: Tsubo exist inside the Tsubo.

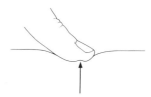

Step 5: Adapt to the ki response.

THIRD ELEMENT
The Ki Method for Super Vessels and Meridians

THE FIVE ASPECTS OF MERIDIAN RECOGNITION

1. Basic knowledge

Taoists in China, and ancient peoples around the world connected to the meridians through their primal sense. Without charts or books to guide them, what they discovered established the system of meridians that can be called basic knowledge. This is the first step in meridian recognition for most people. Some like Master Masunaga are able to go beyond the basic knowledge, as he did to discover the existence of the twelve whole-body meridians. The basic knowledge of Zen Shiatsu was an essential part of his gift to the system of meridians. The ki body meridians of Tao Shiatsu were similarly discovered. The twenty-four meridians (including the sub-meridians), the ring and spiral meridians, and the Super Vessels, were revealed through clinical research and added to the basic knowledge of the meridian system. Seeing meridian streams that have perhaps never been seen and described before brings certain challenges, yet is little in comparison to the contributions of past masters. Taking the subway a few blocks is relatively effortless when you compare it to the work of those who actually built the line piece-by-piece. The work of past masters has made it so much easier for all of us to enter into this stream.

The basic knowledge of the Super Vessels is illustrated in the chart (page 65), which shows where each Super Vessel can be accessed and their range. With a depth of up to seven meters in the ki body, they belong to another dimension of the ki world and are quite unlike the twelve main and sub-meridians. Due to the ki meridian depth, they exhibit a paradoxical nature of also being able to be felt on the surface of the body. Since the giver is able to feel this with the touch sense, Super Vessel recognition is studied at the entrance level. The twelve Super Vessels throughout the body include four that have the sense of being thick, two that are medium-sized, and six that are thin in relation to one another.

Let us take for practice the thick main Super Vessel. It flows a little to the outside of the center on the yang (outward facing) side of the forearm, when the arm is in the position shown (right). It must be remembered that the meridian access line moves by a range of as much as five centimeters when the arm moves through its full range of motion.

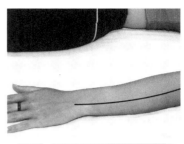
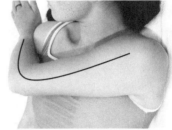
Thick Super Vessel of the arm.

Look at the chart to recognize the basic knowledge—the position of the receiver's body and access location—for the thick main Super Vessel on the arm.

2. Sesshin

Sesshin is the heart state that hopes and prays for the best for others. It is this heart that attracts ki most strongly because it brings relief from over-concern with our own welfare. Separation from others, or continual conflict with them, causes ki to become heavy and rigid. Instead this concern should be directed toward the well-being of others through both the power of the imagination and our actions. Sesshin comes from the language of Japanese Buddhism and describes the heart through which the most positive ki is generated. Universal laws of nature govern the ki world. When ki is given and shared with others without calculation, the peace and relaxation this produces returns to the giver. Tension results in the practice of shiatsu when there are feelings of trying to get something, or to manipulate the ki of others for your own benefit. This tension can be felt physically in the muscles of the giver's upper body. Sesshin gives rise to the healing power of shiatsu: the best outcome for the receiver always arises when the giver's heart prays for the best for the receiver without desire or expectation of benefit or reward. This also returns the best outcome for the giver. Avoiding being too serious about yourself and maintaining a sense of humor is essential to this.

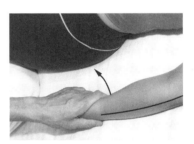
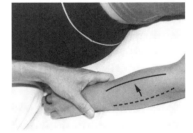
Changing the position of the body changes the location of the Super Vessel.

Living and expressing sesshin is the only way to surpass the conflict of separation that the ego creates between the self and others. The meridians exist only in the state of oneness between giver and receiver. This is neither mere philosophy nor simply an Eastern ideal: it is the nature of the ki world. For thousands of years it has been stated that this cannot be grasped intellectually. The focus of Oriental medicine and shiatsu therapy is the heart itself: it is the way of feeling the receiver's heart as though it were the giver's own.

To see the Super Vessel, express the heart of sesshin toward the receiver, which creates ki unification—the state of oneness of self and others.

3. Inen

Inen means focusing the heart and mind on the meridian, initiating a dialogue with the ki stream of the Super Vessel. The Super Vessel responds to sesshin and inen and reflects in the giver's heart. Try to approach the meridian with the sense of it having a "personality," as it reacts to the attention of empathy. Physical pressure alone closes the ki dimension, and this can become a difficult habit to break.

Direct inen toward the thick main Super Vessel of the forearm and allow nothing else in your mind.

4. Empathetic imagination

Empathetic imagination is the original ki word of Tao Shiatsu and has two aspects: first, imagine *where* the receiver most wants to be pressed, and second, imagine *how* the receiver feels each moment. With the pathway from giver to receiver now activated by inen, you must completely empty your heart and mind, even of inen. Imagine where the receiver most wants to be pressed, with holistic and unconditional acceptance of their life: this gives the receiver's ki complete freedom to express itself. True empathetic imagination exists when the receiver feels this state. The meridian is open and reflects to the giver's heart. Steps one to three above bring us to the point where the location of the meridian is almost clear. Now you need to let go of the previous steps and entrust them to the working of the subconscious. Giving up everything allows the Super Vessel to become completely clear.

Imagine where the receiver wants to be pressed.

5. Naikan

Naikan means to look inward at your heart with moment-to-moment awareness. With the meridian now reflecting to the giver's heart, this is essential. Only by clearly seeing your heart at each moment is the Super Vessel seen.

It exists beyond conflict or separation of giver and receiver. The meridian stream appearing in your heart is without any sense of it being the "other person's meridian." There is only the state of oneness of the object and subject. Seeing the reflection of the meridian in your heart accompanies the feeling of the receiver's life as your own.

With naikan see the Super Vessel reflecting in your heart.

LOCATING MERIDIANS

True study and practice (becoming a student) begins once someone really understands with their heart (and not just their head) that this training follows the law of nature—the Way (道). It may be surprising to hear that it is usually the first time people attempt meridian recognition that they clearly find the location. This happens because at this stage they most fully realize that they do not know anything, so it makes it easier to simply follow the method. Little space exists for the ego to try to rely on self-ability, and most people locate the right place straight away. Then the thinking begins, "How is this happening? Where is the meridian? Is it really here?" and immediately the meridian location is no longer clear.

Following the five aspects is the way to recognize the meridians. Self-ability or reliance on knowledge, such as that written in the classics or books by past masters, cannot recognize the meridians for you. In fact the opposite is true; time and energy will be wasted. The masters of the past saw the meridians through receiving this same heart.

Take the time at the beginning of meridian recognition practice to consciously clear each aspect. This process may require a few seconds for each aspect. However, just like learning to ride a bicycle, in time it becomes a more natural and subconscious process. All five aspects go deeper into the subconscious as meridian recognition continues to be practiced, and they begin to circulate while giving shiatsu. In my experience this circulation is three times per second. The subconscious is deeply engaged and working, even while outwardly it seems as if just a glance at the meridian takes place. Frequent practice, with each stage always being clear, is the basic requirement for training to recognize meridians.

The five aspects are the basis of heart training for all Ki Methods of Tao Shiatsu. Faithfully following these five aspects allows anybody to receive the capacity to locate the meridians precisely. Remember that the meridian chart is just the starting point—the basic knowledge for step one. Even a slightly different body position, from what is shown on the chart, will change the surface location where the meridian can be accessed. All five aspects must be followed for the exact location and depth to be found.

LOCATING THE SUPER VESSEL

1. Follow the five aspects of meridian recognition.
2. Touch with the middle finger.
3. Confirm the location with inen and empathetic imagination, moving the middle finger back and forth. If it is clear, the meridian responds and the receiver clearly feels the giver touching the Super Vessel.

Note: even if the exact physical access location is correct, the Super Vessel will only respond to sesshin heart.

- Next try the same process on the thick Super Vessel of the upper arm (shown on page 87).
- If the meridian location is clear, continue to practice with the other locations shown.

SUPER VESSEL RECOGNITION—PRACTICE LOCATIONS

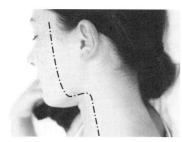
Medium Super Vessel of the neck and face.

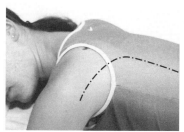
Medium Super Vessel of the shoulder and torso.

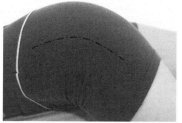
Medium Super Vessel of the hip.

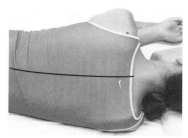
Thick sub Super Vessel of the back.

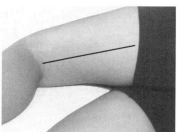
Thick sub Super Vessel of the upper leg.

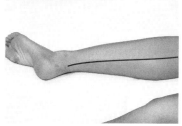
Thick sub Super Vessel of the lower leg.

KI METHOD FOR THE ENTRANCE LEVEL

The Ki Method brings the Super Vessel and the bottom of the kyo meridian together in the ki body. Through unifying and becoming one, jaki is transformed to the positive life-supporting energy of seiki. The Ki Method has three levels. The following explanation is the entrance level method.

KI METHOD FOR SUPER VESSEL TREATMENT

1. Locate the thick Super Vessel on the forearm.
   Imagine where the receiver most wants to be pressed.
   Confirm the tsubo of the Super Vessel with your middle finger.
   Touch the tsubo with your thumb.
2. Find the best angle of your elbow.
3. Lift the thumb off once and then again locate the tsubo with empathetic imagination.
4. Press the tsubo, with deepening empathetic imagination, by straightening the elbow. Let the Super Vessel tsubo reach the bottom of kyo.
5. After a couple of seconds, the Super Vessel will become looser and the rice tip will start to disappear. Relax your elbow, and allow your thumb to come up to the surface.

THE KI METHOD: LEVEL ONE

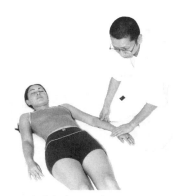
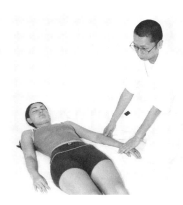

1–2. Find the best angle.

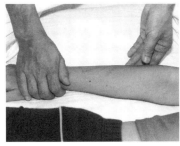
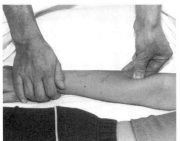
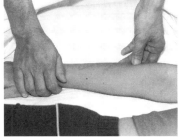

3. Lift your thumb off and locate tsubo again.
4. Press tsubo with empathetic imagination to reach the bottom.
5. Adapt and allow your thumb to come up to the surface.

With practice, it becomes possible to pass over steps 2 and 3. Instead, practice more deeply by imagining the heart and form expressed by the instructor in the photo.

ESSENTIALS OF TREATMENT

FOURTH ELEMENT
Kyo Meridian Treatment

HOW TO PRACTICE KYO MERIDIAN TREATMENT

1. Observe the whole body and imagine the area where the receiver most wants to be pressed.

2. Focus on an area of about fifteen centimeters in diameter.

3. Imagine the line in that area where the receiver most wants to be pressed. This can be a vertical, horizontal, or diagonal line.

4. Allow your subconscious to focus on the point on that line where the receiver most wants to be pressed. Now treat using the Ki Method (see below).
    - The line usually has two to three treatment points along it.
    - When no further points that respond can be found, treatment to this line is finished.

5. Now imagine again where the receiver most wants to be pressed and let your subconscious locate another line in that area.
    - Continue to treat a number of lines in that area. When you cannot locate any further lines that need to be pressed, treatment for that area is finished.
    - Choose another area as in step 1, and then repeat all steps.

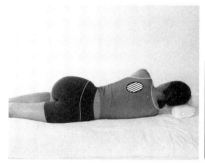

First look at the whole body.

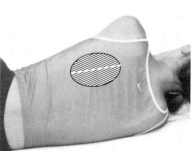

Then focus on the line.

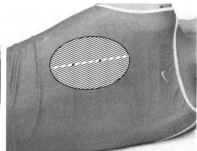

Then on the tsubo.

KI METHOD FOR KYO MERIDIAN TREATMENT

1. a) Touch the tsubo of the kyo line with your center finger and support with your other hand. Press with empathetic imagination to confirm the tsubo is open.

   b) Now touch the tsubo with your thumb, and with increasing empathetic imagination and naikan, slide the thumb back towards the Super Vessel.

   c) It will naturally stop at the Super Vessel, which is about 2–3 mm back from the tsubo. Even though there are numerous Super Vessels, with empathetic imagination your thumb will stop at the most appropriate one.

2. Find the best angle of the elbow (see page 85).

3. Lift your thumb off, and once more locate the Super Vessel with empathetic imagination. Touch again with your thumb.

4. Press the Super Vessel with deepening empathetic imagination, by straightening the elbow. Let the Super Vessel reach the bottom of kyo.

5. After a couple of seconds, the Super Vessel will become looser and the tsubo will start to disappear. Relax your elbow, and allow your thumb to come up to the surface.

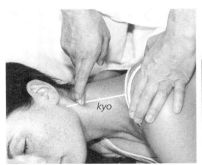
Step 1 a)

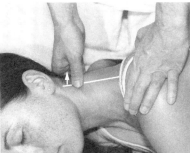
Step 1 b)

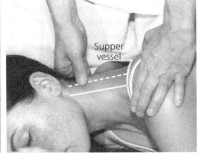
Step 1 c)

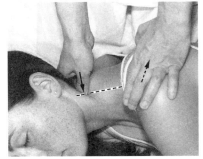
Step 4

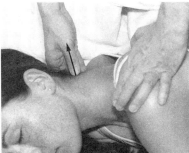
Step 5

ESSENTIALS OF TREATMENT

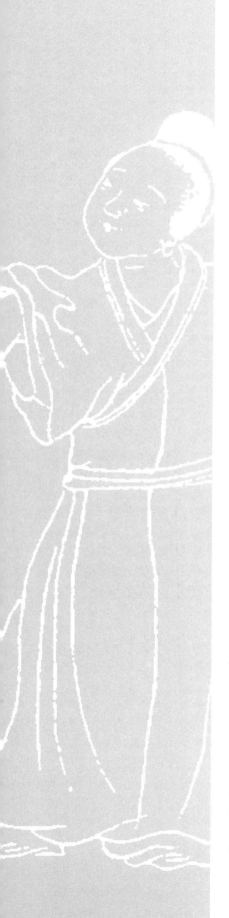

6

TREATING INTERNALIZED KI

SECOND ELEMENT PART TWO
Super Vessel Specific Tsubo (SST)

FROM FOLK REMEDY TO MEDICAL THERAPY

Until Master Masunaga developed the method of diagnosing kyo and jitsu meridians in the hara, shiatsu had been without an established system of meridian diagnosis. In his book *Zen Shiatsu*, Masunaga stated that an established system of diagnosis is what distinguishes a recognized medical therapy from folk remedy. His method gave birth to a new medically therapeutic system centered on ki and meridians. This utilized the uniquely Japanese art of *ampuku*, the practice of palpating the meridians of the abdominal area, or hara. The hara has long held deep significance in Japan as a vital center of awareness in cultural and medical practices.

This system raised a number of difficulties for practice and teaching. How could sho diagnosis be taught as a "method" when it involved the development of the heart state of sesshin? How could people confirm the accuracy of kyo–jitsu diagnosis, when ultimately it did not rely on knowledge or external technique? Master Masunaga sadly passed away before developing a universal system for teaching his method. This helps explain the variety of different forms of diagnosis in Zen Shiatsu today. Simply put, it is not something everyone is able to do.

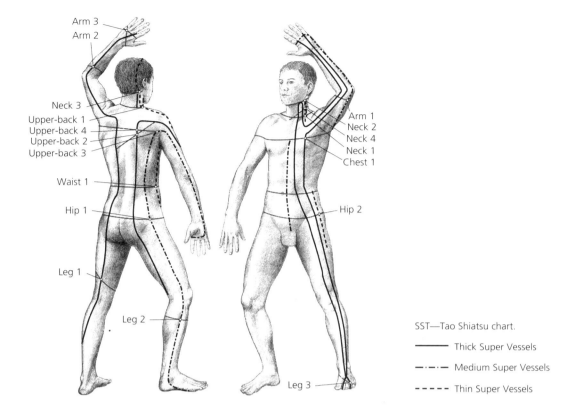

SST—Tao Shiatsu chart.
— Thick Super Vessels
—·—·— Medium Super Vessels
------ Thin Super Vessels

The role of the Super Vessels and the SST (Super Vessel Specific Tsubo) in shiatsu treatment's historical development came about because they helped overcome two great challenges. The first was how to transmit sho diagnosis to others when no teaching method existed. The second was to establish why treatment was no longer proceeding as smoothly and effectively as it had previously, even with correct sho diagnosis. On the surface these challenges seemed unrelated. Yet as it turned out, finding a way to teach diagnosis was also to lead to a solution for the problem of continuing to give effective shiatsu.

EFFECTIVE MEDICAL TREATMENT WITHOUT SHO DIAGNOSIS

Up until 1985, performing hara diagnosis—determining the kyo and jitsu meridians of the abdomen—and then giving shiatsu to the corresponding kyo meridian in the limbs had been very effective. However, this was the turning point in the energetic shift of the meridians and the deepening internalization of kyo, which was occurring as part of the wider changes of the age. The discovery of the Super Vessels and SST resulted from treating the internalized kyo, and led to the creation of Tao Shiatsu. Clinical research revealed twenty-four ki body meridians and the Super Vessels, plus the deeper nature of jaki and the SST to treat it. The changing energetic field of the human body demanded this change in approach to treatment. Previously, shiatsu had involved more conscious awareness of the meridians. The pattern of internalization, however, requires a deep subconscious connection to contact and treat it. The discovery of the Super Vessels created the Ki Method, which unifies the Super Vessels and the bottom of the kyo meridian to heal the internalized distortion. With the Super Vessels, the SST that connects directly to jaki can be treated. This is the source of the kyo meridian and it exists as the deepest level of the ki body.

Shiatsu is entering a new era with the potential for greater effectiveness in treatment of kyo symptoms, and a solution to the dilemma of needing accurate sho diagnosis to give treatment. Discharging and transforming jaki through a safe and effective method has provided real benefits for both the receiver and the giver. Tao Shiatsu's highly evolved meridian system and effective treatment method can be learned without mastery of sho diagnosis. Its teaching system forms a pathway to develop the capacity to see the meridians. This is a system of ki and heart training (*ki shin do*). Its principles and practices develop the heart of sesshin, promoting greater love, understanding, and acceptance of others. In this sense its value is universal, not only for the patients and practitioners of shiatsu.

For the purpose of giving effective treatment in my current clinical practice there is no longer any need to perform sho diagnosis. Sometimes, however, it may prove beneficial to describe to the patient the state of their heart and body through the interpretation offered by sho diagnosis. The healing process of some patients is assisted when they understand more deeply the condition of their heart and body. For example, sho diagnosis may reveal the Gallbladder meridian to be kyo, or deficient in ki. In this case it may be pertinent to ask the patient if their digestion has been troubling them, as Gallbladder kyo leads to difficulty in digesting fat. Another possibility could be that they have a tendency to eat sweets frequently, since the Gallbladder meridian cleans up the toxic effects of white sugar by discharging it through the pattern of Gallbladder kyo. Pointing out the background of the condition can gain the patient's trust that allows deeper treatment, but is not essential for successful treatment. Students attending workshops often increase their trust if they witness clinical demonstrations that reveal the kyo meridian stream when I perform sho diagnosis. This is further strengthened by the opportunity to witness the dramatic improvement in symptoms that comes from giving even a short amount of meridian treatment to a participant. While sho diagnosis may today be helpful in certain situations, however, before Tao Shiatsu it was a necessary part of medical treatment.

Relief from the dilemma of diagnosis

While teaching around the world, I witnessed the wide range of interpretations of the sho diagnosis Master Masunaga practiced. Many different approaches exist, and I came to see that even many teachers of Zen Shiatsu were to some degree "guessing" when they tried to diagnose. Certainly in relation to what Master Masunaga actually taught, there seemed to be an element of grasping in the dark. Ultimately, persisting with such an approach to sho diagnosis will prevent the practitioner's heart from opening to reveal the kyo meridian. There is a fundamental wisdom underlying all existence: when the subconscious is not suppressed, it knows in essence what is true or false. Therefore, this wisdom of the subconscious is betrayed when there are feelings of doubt or uncertainty about the sho diagnosis being taken, especially when this persists over time.

Unification of the conscious mind and the subconscious opens the heart to see ki. Any action that causes separation will hold back the development of this heart state. The establishment of Tao Shiatsu provides the way for anyone wishing to develop their heart to give truly effective medical shiatsu. Ki is purified, and there is relief from the dilemma that sho diagnosis has created. Gone is the necessity of having to hope that the kyo and jitsu diagnosis is more than just a guess.

Heal the source of disease—Treating jaki through SST

SST are special tsubo that enable Tao Shiatsu treatment to be effective without sho diagnosis. These tsubo exist on the Super Vessels, hence their name, with eighteen locations around the body. Working with the SST through the Ki Method is a process of the student shifting from a more conscious and habitual approach, to an increasingly subconscious practice. It is the subconscious work that is the most valuable aspect of this training.

KI METHOD FOR TREATMENT WITH THE EIGHTEEN SST LOCATIONS

Find and treat SST with the Tsubo Method

1. Locate the area in which the SST exists.
   Find the best point in the area by imagining where the receiver most wants to be pressed.
   Treat with the Tsubo Method (see p. 85).

2. Again find the best point in the area and treat.
   Repeat.
   SST usually cannot be located directly with the first point imagined, so repeat and treat three to five points one by one. The SST will then start to echo strongly.

Find and treat SST with Super Vessel recognition

1. All SST are located at points where the Super Vessels cross. For example, Arm SST #2 exists on the thick main Super Vessel of the forearm that was found previously in meridian recognition. In this location is the crossing point of the thick main Super Vessel and the ring Super Vessel, so recognize the Super Vessels following the five aspects.
   - First locate the thick Super Vessel.
   - Next try to see the ring Super Vessel.
   - Then locate the crossing point where the SST exists.

2. The SST exists in that crossing point. However, you cannot locate the SST just from this. The crossing point is about one millimeter in diameter: in that one millimeter try to imagine the place the receiver most wants to be pressed. The empathy expressed through sesshin by the giver causes the tsubo to respond, making it possible to locate the SST. SST can be felt as a larger rice tip than that of regular tsubo.

3. After locating the SST, treat by following the steps for the Tsubo Method.

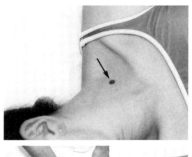

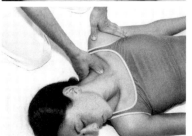

THE EIGHTEEN SST LOCATIONS

1. At the base of the neck, with the receiver lying on their back with their head turned away from the side being treated. The *ho* (supporting) hand is placed on the shoulder or upper arm, and the *sha* (projecting) direction of the thumb is inward, toward the trachea (airway).

   Jaki is discharged from the chest or the throat. Usually the echo travels to the upper arm and then to the forearm and toward the fingertips.

2. In the upper front area of the neck, with the receiver lying in the side or face-up position (as above). The giver kneels side-on to the receiver with one or both knees down. The giver's ho hand is placed on the head or shoulder and the sha direction of the thumb is toward the inside

center of the head. The thumb joint can be bent if necessary.

The echo travels toward the ears and the inside of the eyes. In addition to the fingertips and feet, the cavities in the skull are also locations through which jaki is discharged. This SST can be especially effective in cases where SST #3 on the neck is closed, due to the deep internalization of jaki.

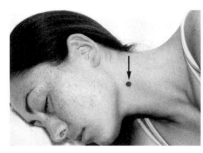
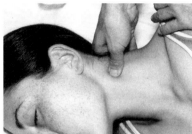

3. In the upper area of the back of the neck, with the receiver lying in the side position. The giver kneels side-on to the receiver with one or both knees down. The ho hand is placed on the shoulder and the sha direction of the thumb is toward the inside center of the head.

   The echo usually moves to the eyes, ears, mouth, and sometimes to the top of the head. Jaki is generally released from the head.

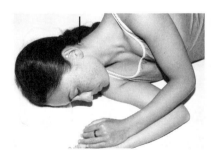
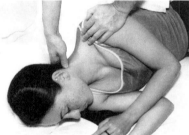

4. On the neck between SST #1 and #2 on the spiral (diagonal) Super Vessel, with the receiver lying in the side position. The giver's ho hand

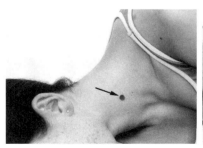
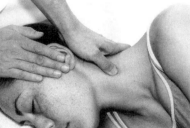

is placed on the head and the sha direction of the thumb is toward the inside of the torso around the middle *danchu* tanden, located between the nipples in the center of the chest.

Jaki from the chest is released toward the arm.

5. At the base of the neck or top of the shoulder, with the receiver lying in the side position. The giver's ho hand is placed on the shoulder or head and the sha direction of the thumb is toward the inside of the hara (abdomen).

    If the echo is toward the scapula, the location and method are correct. Sometimes the echo is to the head, but this indicates either that the depth of the method was a little shallow, or that the location was not exactly on the SST.

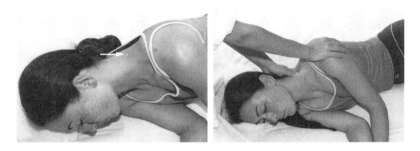

6. In the upper part of the back, slightly away from the spine, with the receiver in the side position. Use both hands in the butterfly position, where one thumb acts as ho, and the other works on the SST as sha. The sha direction of the thumb is inside the shoulder blade.

    The echo is toward the outside of the shoulder and down into the arm.

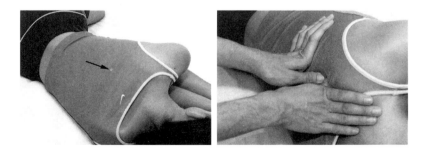

7. At the top of the upper arm on the outside of the shoulder, with the receiver in the side position. The giver faces the receiver. Use both

hands in the butterfly position. The sha direction of the thumb is toward the center of the shoulder blade.

The echo travels through the whole arm. Jaki is discharged from both the shoulder and back. This SST is especially effective for treating shoulder stiffness. It is important not to forget to work on the arm after this SST, in order to avoid a strong Menken Response after treatment. Note: the Menken Response may manifest itself following therapy, when the expulsion of energy toxins in the form of jaki leads to the surfacing of emotions and ailments that had been previously suppressed. Symptoms such as fatigue, drowsiness, diarrhea, headache, or increased pain may arise. Providing adequate treatment to the limbs decreases the severity of the Menken Response.

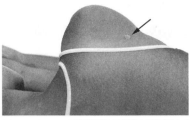
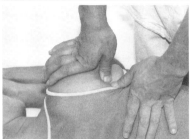

8. On the back close to SST #6 but slightly higher, with the receiver in the sitting position. The ho hand is placed on the shoulder and the sha direction of the thumb is toward the center of the chest.

   After giving whole body treatment, jaki may come up from deep inside to the surface and remain in the upper back area. This SST is very useful in alleviating this situation and is therefore usually worked on toward the end of the treatment.

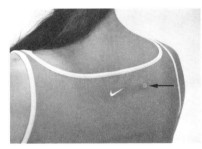
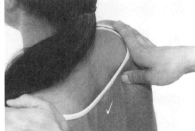

9. On the upper inner arm, approximately two-fifths of the distance from the elbow to the armpit, with the receiver lying on their back. The ho

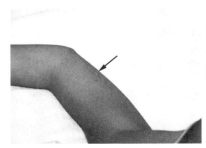
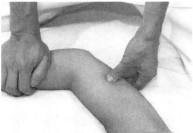

hand is placed on the lower arm, and the sha direction of the thumb is inside the arm and slightly toward the elbow.

The echo travels down the whole arm and into the hand, with jaki discharged through the fingers.

10. On the outer forearm, with the receiver lying on their back. The ho hand is placed on the receiver's hand, and the sha direction of the thumb is inside the arm.

    The echo is felt into the hand and fingertips, and may sometimes include discharge of jaki from the spiral meridian. The finger or fingers affected are not always the same.

    Jaki discharged from the torso during treatment may accumulate here, or in the upper arm, sometimes creating numbness or a dull sensation. Pain in the arm in the days following treatment can also occur. Treating this SST is important to protect against jaki build-up, leading to increased manifestation of the Menken Response.

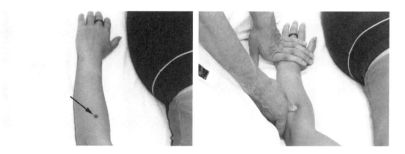

11. On the back of the hand, in the space between the little and ring finger bones, with the receiver lying face up. The ho hand is placed on the wrist and the sha direction of the thumb is toward the inside of the hand's centerline.

    The echo is usually felt in the fingertips, but may also be felt in the arm when jaki stuck in the upper arm discharges through the fingertips.

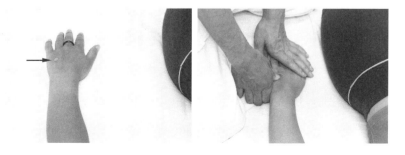

12. On the chest, at the midpoint along the line from the nipple to the collarbone, with the receiver lying face up and their neck turned away from the side receiving treatment. The ho hand is placed on the upper arm and the sha direction of the thumb is inside the center of the chest.

    The echo travels out through the upper arm and discharges jaki from the chest. It may also release tension of the face and allow breathing to become deeper and more relaxed.

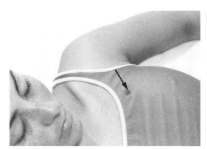 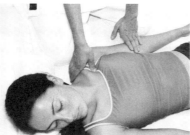

13. On the lower back, between the ribs and the hip, with the receiver lying on their side. The giver kneels beside the receiver with their outside knee raised. The ho hand is placed on the lower back, and the sha direction of the thumb is toward the spine. When this SST is located correctly, the receiver has the sensation of it being between the muscle and the spine.

    This SST exists at a very deep level and releases jaki from the abdomen. The echo goes toward the hip and lower leg.

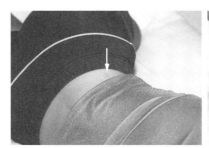 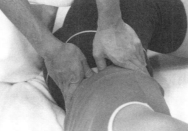

14. At the base of the depression on the hipbone, with the receiver in the side position. The giver faces the receiver's abdomen and uses the butterfly position of the hands. The hand closest to the waist is the ho hand, and the sha direction of the thumb is toward the center of the lower abdomen.

Jaki is discharged from the whole of the lower back. Usually it echoes first in the upper leg, and then toward the lower leg and toes.

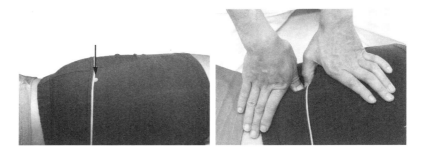

15. In the depressed area at the top of the leg where it meets the pelvic bone, with the receiver lying face up. The knee of the leg being treated is raised and moved across toward the other leg. The ho hand supports the knee, and the sha direction is toward the lower abdomen. The ho hand moves the leg back toward the giver, synchronized with the application of pressure by the sha thumb.

The echo is usually strong in the leg. When jaki from the lower back is deeply internalized, it goes into the front of the hip and pelvis. This means SST #14 will be closed, while this SST becomes active.

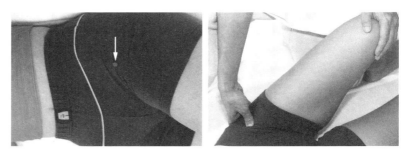

16. On the back of the upper leg, a little outside from the centerline, and about one-third of the distance between the knee and the buttock–leg

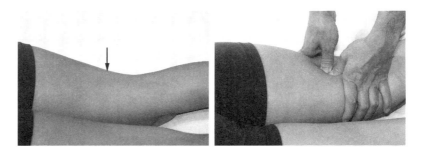

crease, with the receiver in the face-down position. The giver uses the butterfly position of the hands with one thumb as ho and the sha direction of the other thumb toward the center of the leg, angled slightly toward the lower back.

The echo moves down the leg toward the foot, and jaki is released from the torso.

17. On the outside and middle of the lower leg, with the knee of the leg being treated bent outward, and the receiver in the side position. This brings the SST to the most treatable position, where it may almost appear to be on the bone.

    The echo is in the upper leg or outside of the foot, and sometimes both at the same time. Jaki that is stuck in the upper leg is able to start moving toward the toes.

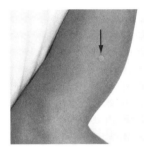 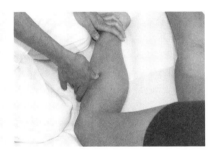

18. On the top of the foot, between the fourth and fifth toes, the receiver in the face-up position with the leg being treated bent so that the sole of the foot is on the ground. The ho hand is placed on the toes and the sha direction of the thumb is toward the inside of the foot.

    The echo is toward and into the toes. When jaki moves toward the extremities, it is not always fully discharged. Sometimes it remains stuck in the joint. With this SST, jaki that is stuck around the ankle, or remaining in the leg from the treatment, can be released.

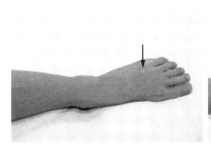 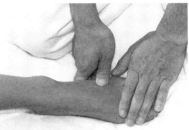

7

WHOLE BODY KI MERIDIAN SHIATSU

FIFTH ELEMENT
Basic Form

BASIC FORM SUPPORTS THE KYO DEFICIENCY OF KI

Tao Shiatsu classes and seminars involve the study of its Five Elements. In all of the three levels that comprise Tao Shiatsu practitioner training, each element is studied in turn following a specific order, or circulation. Chapters four, five, and six explained the first four elements—Ki Doin, tsubo and SST treatment, Super Vessel recognition with Ki Method treatment, and kyo meridian treatment. The last element to be studied is Basic Form treatment, which will be explained in this chapter. In Basic Form, treatment is given to the receiver following a specific sequence: the areas of the body treated, the order they are treated in, and the Super Vessels used, are all predetermined. Four positions are utilized, with the receiver lying on their side, face-down, face-up, and sitting, and these are known as the Basic Forms. The time required to give all the forms consecutively ranges from forty to sixty minutes, depending on the practitioner's experience. At the third level an advanced Basic Form is taught, which is based on a unique approach of supporting the hara throughout the form. With the receiver lying on their side, the giver places one knee under the patient's hip and the other knee under the armpit to support the body. This form takes fifteen to twenty minutes. It would seem to make sense that the Basic Form study would come at the beginning of training, but in Tao Shiatsu it is taught last. This is because almost all of the preceding elements of study are involved: the Tsubo Method, Super Vessel recognition, and kyo meridian treatment. This makes the Ki Method for the Basic Form the most challenging element to master.

The clinical practice of Tao Shiatsu is centered on Basic Form and kyo meridian treatment. All Oriental medical treatment is based on the principles of *hoho ki* (ki supporting method) and *shaho ki* (ki projecting method). In shiatsu, hoho ki—the supporting method—is traditionally understood to mean filling up the ki that has become deficient, while shaho ki—the projecting method—shifts and transfers excessive ki. For Tao Shiatsu treatment, the purpose of hoho ki is to change jaki into seiki, allowing ki to be replenished and revitalized. Basic Form treatment achieves this. Shaho ki relieves jaki by expelling ki toxins from the body, which is achieved through kyo meridian treatment. In cases where the patient is experiencing acute pain, kyo meridian treatment is performed first to relieve the symptoms, followed by the Basic Form treatment. In cases of chronic pain, or for general treatment, the Basic Form treatment is performed first, followed by kyo meridian treatment.

KI METHOD FOR THE BASIC FORMS

Each Basic Form sequence determines the Super Vessels to be used and the number of tsubo on each Super Vessel to be treated. Basic Form treatment has its own Ki Method, which is characterized by the giver's action of "taking up the slack" of the receiver's body. In practical terms, this involves moving the skin and muscle with a forward and downward motion at an angle of about 45 degrees. A corresponding shift takes place in the ki body to release and channel ki. This method contrasts with the direct downward pressure applied perpendicularly to the surface of the body, traditionally used in shiatsu. The ki direction to take up the slack of the skin is depicted in all of the following photos for the side position Basic Form practice. All Basic Forms of Tao Shiatsu use the following Ki Method.

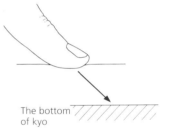

Press at an angle of about 45°.

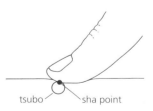

The sha (ki concentrated) point connects to the tsubo.

How to practice the Ki Method for Basic Form treatment

1. Locate the Super Vessel and tsubo

Check and confirm the Super Vessel to be used and how many tsubo on the Super Vessel are to be treated.

Say the words "sha point to Super Vessel." Then slide the sha point of the part of the body (thumb, elbow, or knee) being used to treat until it naturally stops.

- Ki and meridians respond to both words and images, meaning the sha point will naturally stop at the Super Vessel. If you try consciously to find the Super Vessel, it will not happen. Trust the method and leave the doing up to Tao: with this heart the method works and the sha point will naturally stop.

- The sha point is the place where ki concentrates most. It is not a physical point but an expression of ki. Remember, this method of shiatsu is not about simply applying physical pressure with a particular part of the body.

After locating the Super Vessel, again say "sha point to Super Vessel." Slide the sha point along the Super Vessel. The same principle applies and the sha point naturally stops at the tsubo to be treated.

In Level One, it is especially important to have faith in the method, as this will develop the necessary heart of entrusting "the doing" to Tao.

2. Find the best angle of the elbow

Finding the best angle of the elbow for the sha point of the thumb or hand has already been explained in the Tsubo Method section.

- When the sha point is the elbow (on the ulna bone of the forearm), there are three movements to find the best angle: sideways, tilting up and down, and rotating around the middle finger (photos below).

- When the sha point is the knee (on the tibia bone, just below the knee), there is only the tilting up-and-down movement to find the best angle.

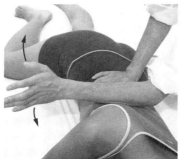
Tilting up and down.

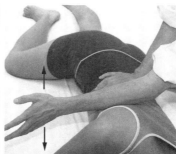
Sideways.

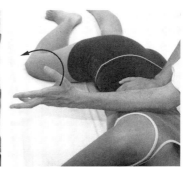
Rotating around the middle finger.

After a certain level of empathetic imagination is reached, the best angle will be taken subconsciously.

3. Locate the tsubo again

Come off the tsubo once and locate it again by imagining where within the tsubo the receiver most wants to be pressed. This is explained in detail in the Tsubo Method section.

This gives the best sha point connection to the Super Vessel tsubo.

4. Reach the bottom of the tsubo with empathetic imagination

When using the sha point of the thumb, press the Super Vessel tsubo with empathetic imagination as you straighten your elbow and take up slack of the receiver's skin.

- When using the sha point of the elbow: raise the hand so that the sha point moves downward to reach the depth.
- When using the sha point of the knee: raise the hip to reach the depth.

5. Adaptation

Keep increasing empathetic imagination at the bottom for 1–2 seconds. Then relax your elbow and let the thumb come up to the surface, synchronized with your imagination.

- When using the sha point of the elbow: lower the hand.
- When using the sha point of the knee: lower the hip.

HOW TO PRACTICE BASIC FORM TREATMENT USING THE IMAGE OF THE TEACHER

1. Look at each photo and then copy the movement.
2. Not only follow the physical form and position shown in each photograph, but also deeply imagine the form and expression of the heart with which the teacher is giving shiatsu.
3. The Super Vessel tsubo will reach the bottom of tsubo through the ki and heart received from the teacher.

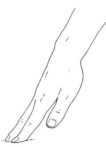

Grasping pressure

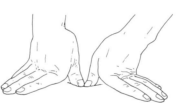

Palm pressure

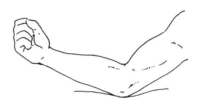

Heel of the hand pressure

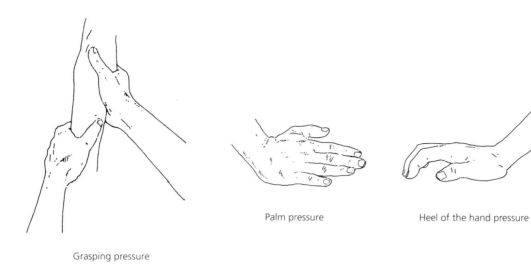

Four finger pressure

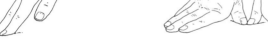

Thumb pressure

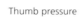

Elbow (ulna) pressure

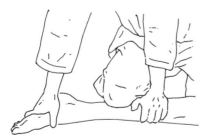

Knee pressure

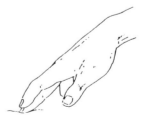

Center finger pressure

Techniques for Basic Form shiatsu.

Basic Form in the Side Position

All Super Vessels for Basic Form are shown on the chart as follows:
Thick = ——— Medium = –·–·– Thin = ············
Place the receiver in the position shown in the photo and take the position shown for the giver.

- Sha (projecting) hand position and ki direction is shown as a solid line with the arrow showing the direction to take up slack. →

- Ho (supporting) hand position and ki direction is shown as a broken line with the arrow showing the direction to take up slack. ⇢

Begin with the receiver lying on his or her right side, and the head supported by a pillow. The giver positions him or herself behind the receiver, facing their legs. Kneel with the balls of the feet touching the ground and the toes up.

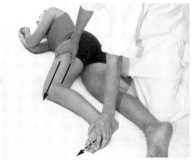

1. GRASPING PRESSURE TO THE LEFT THIGH

HO: Hold the foot with your left hand. Direction of taking up slack is toward the toes.
SUPER VESSEL: Thick main, located on the inside of the leg.
SHA: Place the right hand on the upper leg, with the sha point of the thumb on the Super Vessel. Take up slack toward the knee on three points.

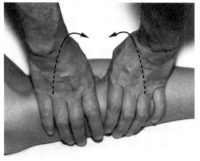

2. THUMB PRESSURE TO THE CALF

HO: Place both hands together evenly on the lower leg. The direction of taking up slack is toward you, through rotating your hands backward.
SUPER VESSEL: Thick main (located on the inside of the leg).
SHA: Place the sha point of your right thumb on the Super Vessel and take up slack toward you at three points.

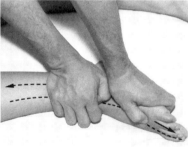

3. GRASPING PRESSURE TO THE OUTSIDE OF THE FOOT.

HO: Place your right hand on the lower leg above the ankle. The direction of taking up slack is toward the knee.
SUPER VESSEL: Thin main (located in the center of the foot).
SHA: Grasp the foot with your left hand so the sha point of the thumb is on the Super Vessel. Take up slack in the direction of the toes on three points. Start from above the toes and move toward the ankle.

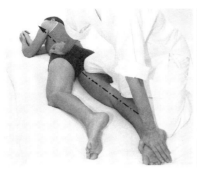
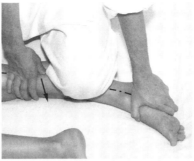
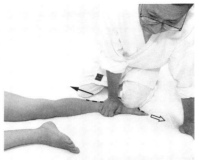

4. KNEE PRESSURE TO THE INNER THIGH OF THE UPPER LEG.

HO: Place your left hand on the bottom of the receiver's right foot and your right hand on the buttock. Take up slack toward the back with your left hand, and simultaneously toward the toes with your right hand.

SUPER VESSEL: Medium (located in the center of the leg).

SHA: Place the sha point of your right knee on the Super Vessel of the upper leg. Take up slack toward the receiver's other leg on three points.

5. KNEE PRESSURE TO THE LOWER LEG

HO: Hold the bottom of the receiver's foot with your left hand. The direction of taking up slack is toward the toes. Place your right knee on the upper leg, close to the buttock. The direction of taking up slack is toward the buttock.

SUPER VESSEL: Medium, located in the center of the leg.

SHA: The sha point of your right thumb is placed on the Super Vessel of the lower leg. Take up slack on three points toward the other leg. The left knee is placed next to the thumb and supports it, but gives no downward pressure.

• Move down toward the foot.

6. KNEE PRESSURE TO THE BOTTOM OF THE FOOT

HO: Place your right hand on the lower leg above the ankle. The direction of taking up slack is toward the knee. The left hand is placed on the floor.

SUPER VESSEL: Thin sub in the center of the foot.

SHA: The sha point of your left knee is placed on the Super Vessel. Take up slack in the direction of the toes on three points. Start from the heel and move toward the toes.

• Kneel parallel to the receiver with your right knee raised. Let your left leg lightly touch the receiver's back.

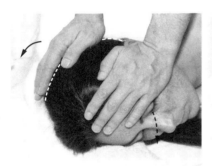
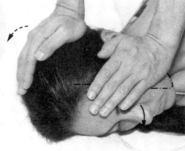
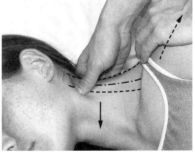

7. PALM PRESSURE TO THE BACK OF THE HEAD

HO: Place your left palm around the receiver's temple area. Direction of taking up slack is outward toward the face, with a spiral movement.

SUPER VESSEL: Thin main.

SHA: The sha point of the heel of your right hand is placed on the Super Vessel. Take up slack in an outward direction on three points, with a spiral movement.

8. PALM PRESSURE TO THE SIDE OF THE FACE

HO: Place your right palm on the back of the receiver's head. Direction of taking up slack is outward, with a spiral movement

SUPER VESSEL: Medium.

SHA: The sha point of the heel of your left hand is placed on the Super Vessel. Take up slack in an outward direction on three points, with a spiral movement.

• Move down slightly to work on the neck

9. GRASPING PRESSURE TO THE NECK

HO: Place your left hand on the top of the receiver's shoulder. Direction of taking up slack is back and slightly toward you.

SUPER VESSEL: Thin sub (inside neck), medium (center), thin main (outside neck).

SHA: Place the sha point of your right thumb on the first Super Vessel. Take up slack on three points on each of the three Super Vessels, by rotating your hand away from you.

• Drop your right knee down and sit on your heels with the toes up.

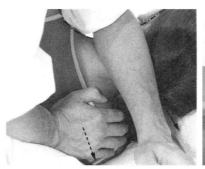
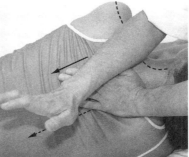
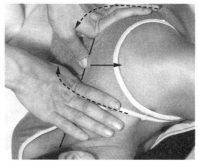

10. ULNA PRESSURE TO THE NECK

HO: Place your right hand on the receiver's right (lower) shoulder blade. Direction of taking up slack is downward.
SUPER VESSEL: Medium (center).
SHA: Place the sha point on the ulna bone of the forearm on the Super Vessel. Take up slack outward on three points.

- Move around to face the receiver's head. Sit on your heels with the toes up.

11. ULNA PRESSURE TO THE TOP OF THE SHOULDER

HO: Place your left hand on the receiver's back. Direction of taking up slack is toward the feet.
SUPER VESSEL: Thin (flowing across the top of the shoulder).
SHA: Place the sha point on the ulna bone of the forearm on the Super Vessel. Take up slack toward the feet on three points.

- Move around and face the receiver's upper back. Sit on your heels with the toes up.

12A. THUMB PRESSURE TO THE UPPER BACK

HO: Place your hands on the receiver's back in the butterfly position. Take up slack by drawing the fingers back toward you while pressing the thumbs forward.
SUPER VESSEL: Thick sub (slightly outside from the left side of the spine).
SHA: The sha point of the right thumb takes up slack at three points on the Super Vessel away from the giver.

- Move down to the lower back and sit on your heels parallel to the receiver. Raise your right (outside) knee and let your left leg (toe up) lightly touch the receiver's back.

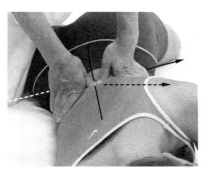
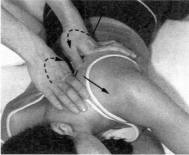
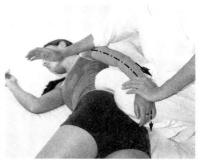

12B. THUMB PRESSURE TO THE LOWER BACK

HO: Place the whole of your left hand around the waist, above the receiver's spine. The direction of taking up slack is away from you.
SUPER VESSEL: Thick sub (just out from the left side of the receiver's spine).
SHA: Place the sha point of your right thumb on the Super Vessel above the spine, with your fingers below on the other side of spine. Take up slack on three points away from you.

- Move up to face the receiver's shoulder. Sit on your heels with the toes up.

12C. THUMB PRESSURE TO THE INSIDE OF THE SHOULDER BLADE

HO: Place your hands on the receiver's back in the butterfly position. Take up slack by drawing the fingers back toward you, while pressing the thumbs forward.
SUPER VESSEL: Thick main (slightly inside from the edge of the shoulder blade).
SHA: The sha point of the right thumb takes up slack at three points on the Super Vessel away from the giver.

- Rest on the balls of your feet, raise both knees and rest them lightly on the receiver's waist and buttock. Keep the weight on your feet and try not to lean on the receiver.

13. ULNA PRESSURE TO THE ARM

HO: Place the receiver's left arm on your knees and hold the wrist with your left hand. The direction of taking up slack is toward the receiver's hand.
SUPER VESSEL: Thin sub (around the center of the arm).
SHA: Place the sha point (on the ulna bone) of the forearm on the Super Vessel. Take up slack toward the hand on three points of the upper arm, and three points of the lower arm.

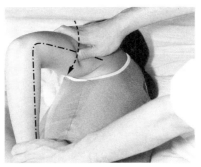 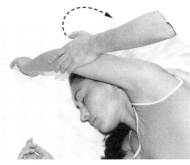

14A. GRASPING PRESSURE TO THE ARM

HO: Bend the receiver's arm, place the back of the hand on the waist and hold their wrist with your left hand. The direction of taking up slack is back toward you by rotating your hand.
SUPER VESSEL: Medium.
SHA: Grasp the upper arm and place the sha point of your right thumb on the Super Vessel. Take up slack toward you at three points, by rotating your hand inward.

14B. GRASPING PRESSURE TO THE ARM

HO: Keep your right hand at the last point of the upper arm, it now becomes the ho. The direction of taking up slack is toward you, by rotating your hand.
SUPER VESSEL: Medium.
SHA: Grasp the lower arm below the elbow and place the sha point of your left thumb on the Super Vessel. Take up slack toward you at three points, by rotating your hand inward.

- Now turn, while still holding the receiver's arm above the elbow with your left hand, and sit on your heels (toes up) parallel to the receiver. Lightly touch the receiver's back with your left leg.

15. ROTATING THE ARM AND SHOULDER

HO: Place your right hand on the shoulder blade and use this as the pivot of movement.
SHA: With your left arm cupping the upper arm above the elbow, take up slack outward toward the elbow and rotate the arm in a clockwise motion three times. On the third rotation, bring the arm down and place it on the head.

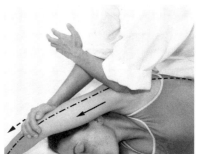 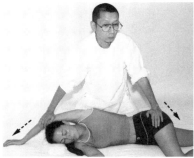 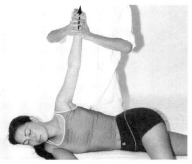

16. ULNA PRESSURE TO THE INSIDE OF THE UPPER ARM

HO: Hold the receiver's arm on or below the elbow. The direction of taking up slack is toward the receiver's hand.
SUPER VESSEL: Medium.
SHA: The giver's left arm is perpendicular to the receiver's arm. Place the sha point of the ulna on the first point (in the depression just below the shoulder bone) and take up slack toward the elbow. Then on three points on the Super Vessel of the upper arm.

- Turn and face the receiver with your hips raised.

17A. ARM EXTENSIONS

Place your right arm on the arm above the elbow and your left arm on the hip. By leaning your body weight, take up slack in an outward direction with both hands simultaneously.

17B. ARM EXTENSIONS

Take the receiver's left wrist and hold it with interlaced fingers against your body. Then, by leaning your upper body backward, take up slack on the arm. Once only. Place the arm down gently.

- Turn and place yourself parallel to the receiver. Sit on your left heel (with toes down) and raise the right knee. Lightly touch the receiver back with your left leg.

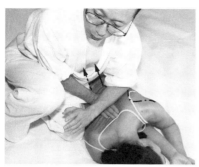 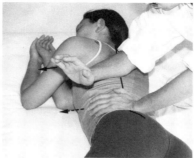 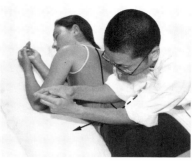

18. ULNA PRESSURE TO THE BACK

HO: The right palm is placed near the sha point of the ulna and moves with it. The direction of taking up slack is toward the hip.
SUPER VESSEL: Medium.
SHA: The sha point of the giver's left ulna is placed on the Super Vessel. Take up slack toward the waist on three points, starting from the lower part of the shoulder blade. Continue on three points from the waist to the buttocks.

• Turn and face the receiver's back.

19A. ELBOW/ ULNA PRESSURE TO THE BACK

HO: The left hand is placed on the waist. The direction of taking up slack is away from you.
SUPER VESSEL: Thick sub.
SHA: Place the sha point of your left ulna on the Super Vessel. Take up slack away from you on three points, moving from the shoulder blade to the middle of the back.

19B. ELBOW/ ULNA PRESSURE TO THE BACK

HO AND SHA: As above.
SUPER VESSEL: Thick main (just inside the inner edge of the shoulder blade).

• Move further down toward the receiver's hips.

20. ELBOW PRESSURE TO THE LOWER BACK

HO: Place your left ulna on the hip. Interlace the hands with your fingers inside and the tips of the index fingers touching. Cross the left thumb over the top of the right. The direction of taking up slack is away from you.
SUPER VESSEL: Thick sub.
SHA: Place the sha point of your right ulna on the Super Vessel and take up slack away from you. Treat four or five points, from the lower back and continuing to the upper sacrum, gradually bringing both elbows together.

• Kneel outside the receiver's right leg, or between the two legs depending on the relative sizes of giver and receiver. Position your left leg perpendicular to the upper left leg of the receiver.

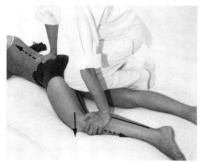 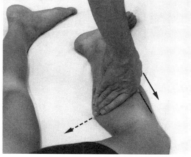

21. KNEE PRESSURE TO THE THIGH

HO: Place your right hand on the patient' hip. Your left hand is placed on the receiver's left leg below the knee. The direction of taking up slack is toward the foot.
SUPER VESSEL: Thick main.
SHA: The sha point of the giver's left knee is placed on the Super Vessel and takes up slack on three points downward.

• Move downward and face the lower leg.

22. THUMB PRESSURE TO THE LOWER LEG

HO: Place both hands together, with the thumbs on the front of the leg and the fingers providing supporting pressure behind. The direction of taking up slack is back toward the other leg.
SUPER VESSEL: Thick main.
SHA: Place the sha point of the giver's right thumb on the Super Vessel and take up slack on three points down toward the floor.

23. REPEAT STEP 3 ON THE FOOT.

Then repeat steps 4, 5 and 6 on the inner leg.

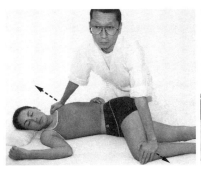 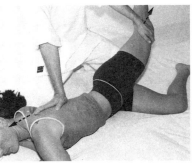 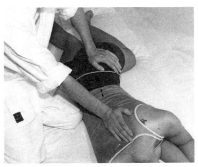

24. SPINAL STRETCH

Position yourself perpendicular to the patient with your hips raised.

- Place your right hand on the left shoulder area (toward the underarm) and take up slack to move the shoulder in the direction of the floor.
- Place your left hand above the patient's knee and take up slack simultaneously in the opposite direction to your right hand.

25. SIDE STRETCH

With your left hand, pick up the receiver's left leg. Place your left knee against the back of the upper thigh, near the buttock. Now place your right hand on the receiver's right shoulder blade. The direction of taking up slack is toward the head. Draw the leg back by taking up slack toward the toes and using the knee as a pivot.

- Sit on your heels (with toes up) beside the receiver.

26. COMPLETION—BRING KI DOWN AND BRUSH OFF

HO: Place your left hand on the patient's lower back.

SHA: Give palm pressure with the right hand to three points on the left side of the spine. Take up slack toward the feet simultaneously with both hands and bring ki down.

- Place the right hand at one location, on or near the shoulder bade. Take up slack downward and release, brushing the hand with increasing speed down the back to the hip and off. Do twice.

Repeat steps 1–26 on the opposite side.

HOW TO DEVELOP A PROGRAM OF FIVE ELEMENTS STUDY

Studying with a Tao Shiatsu teacher is, of course, the best opportunity to master these methods for giving treatment. However, when this is not possible the following guidelines will provide you with a way of studying Tao Shiatsu, especially by using the image of the teacher as described earlier. Tsubo Method and Ki Method training *must* be completed before giving treatment.

Follow this program:

1. Practice Renki (p. 76) and Ki Breathing (p. 123).

2. Practice tsubo and SST location and treatment, with both the Tsubo Method and the Ki Method (see next page).

3. Learn and practice all the Basic Form treatment positions. Only the side position is shown in this book. For photos and explanations of the face-down, face-up, and sitting positions see *Tao Shiatsu: Life Medicine for the 21st Century*.

4. For giving treatment, perform Basic Form treatment in the side position, and then follow with meridian treatment.

NOTE: The clinical practice, and teaching of the Tao Shiatsu methods, can only be carried out by people who have been certified by the International Tao Shiatsu Society.

TREATING TSUBO WITH THE TSUBO METHOD

1. Locate the rice tip and continue to feel it each moment as the tsubo goes toward the bottom, reaches the bottom, and ki begins to press back against your thumb.
2. Keep empathetically imagining the receiver's life sensation at each moment.
3. Adapt to the receiver's ki and relax your elbow when the bottom of the tsubo starts coming up.

Work with these steps and then practice with the Ki Method.

TREATING TSUBO WITH THE KI METHOD

1. Locate the tsubo with empathetic imagination and confirm with your middle finger.
2. Touch the tsubo with your thumb, and with increasing empathetic imagination and naikan (focusing the mind and heart toward the Super Vessel) slide your thumb back toward the Super Vessel.
3. Your thumb will naturally stop at the Super Vessel, which is about 2–3 mm back from the tsubo. Even though a number of Super Vessels will exist in any area, empathetic imagination will allow the most appropriate one for the tsubo to be selected.

Follow the Ki Method to let the Super Vessel tsubo reach the bottom of kyo by straightening your elbow.

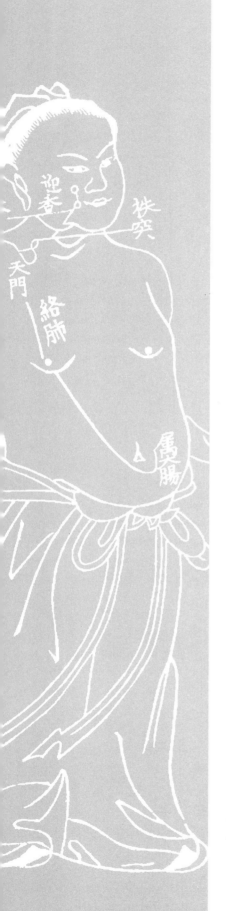

8

SHIATSU SELF-TREATMENT METHOD

Of course, the most effective way to receive treatment is from a Tao Shiatsu practitioner. However, this is not always possible, and so this chapter explains how to give self-treatment. Practice all of the Renki exercises (see p. 76) and Ki Breathing meditation (p. 123) daily. This is highly recommended. Even after just a few weeks of practice you will feel the difference it makes to your ki.

If you have any pain or symptoms, you can treat yourself with the method shown in the following pages. The tsubo that will be treated are the SST that were studied in chapter six. However, it is not possible to self-treat all of these areas, so only fourteen points are suggested here.

Tao Shiatsu teaches how to find tsubo by empathetic imagination. It is possible to direct this feeling toward yourself and imagine where you most want to be pressed in a given area. Just look for a few seconds at the selected area, and imagine where you most want to be pressed. The tsubo's response will be felt. Touch the place with your middle finger and press to see if you feel any echo. If the tsubo echoes, then press with the sha point of the thumb (use finger or knuckle if thumb is not possible) and imagine the bottom of the tsubo. Repeat on the same tsubo two or three times until the echo changes or lessens. Repeat this process two or three times on different tsubo in the same area.

It is very important that you follow the same order as shown here, and continue to treat until the symptom changes. This may require continuing with treatment on a daily basis.

METHOD FOR SELF-SHIATSU

1. Locate the area of the tsubo.
2. Look at the area for a few seconds and imagine where you most need to be pressed within a circle of 3–4 cm diameter.
3. The tsubo will respond, giving you a sense of its location.
4. Touch this location with your middle finger, and check for an echo. Start again if there is no echo.
5. If there is an echo, press the tsubo with the sha point and imagine it reaching the bottom. Come back up when the echo becomes less or the tsubo starts to disappear.
6. Repeat this two or three times until the echo is much less, or disappears altogether.
7. Repeat steps 2 to 6 on another two or three tsubo in the same area.
8. Move to the next area.

This treatment is good for a variety of symptoms. Practicing regularly, or even daily, will change the condition of both heart and body. If for any reason you cannot give treatment to all of the tsubo recommended, then focus on the tsubo in the area of the symptom you suffer from (if it is accessible to self-treatment). In any case, always try to treat the upper body tsubo in particular.

The most effective treatment is when, as you press the tsubo, you imagine you are treating the pain and suffering of all human beings, rather than just your own (do not forget to include the people *you do not like* as well as those you do!). Try it and feel the difference it makes. You will be surprised.

UPPER BODY SST POINTS

Point numbers refer to the Tao Shiatsu SST chart (see p. 95).

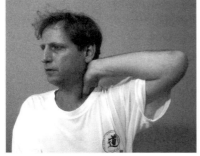

Neck #1

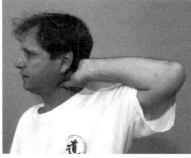

Neck #2

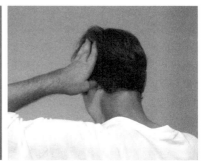

Neck #3

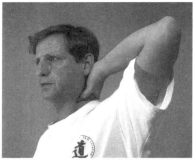
Neck #4

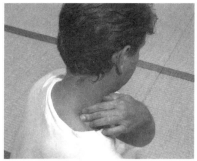
Upper Back #1

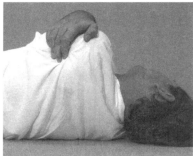
Upper Back #2

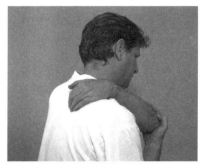
Upper Back #3

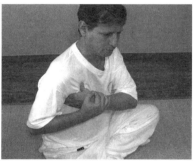
Chest #1

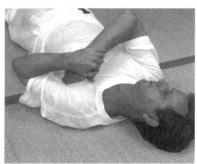
Chest #2

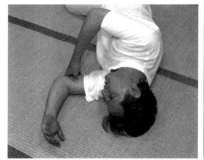
Arm #1

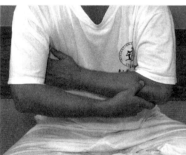
Arm #2

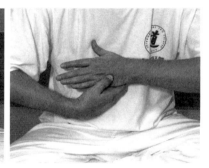
Arm #3

Repeat the same tsubo on the other side.

LOWER BODY SST POINTS

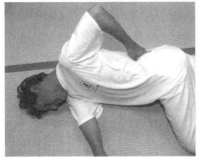
Waist #1

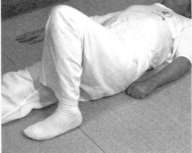
Hip #1

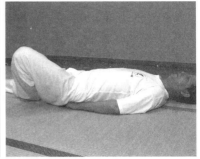
Hip #2

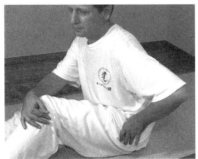
Hip #3

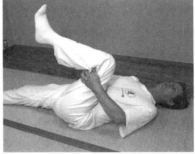
Leg #1

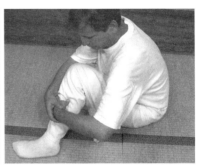
Leg #2

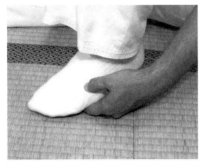
Leg #3

Repeat the same tsubo on the other side.

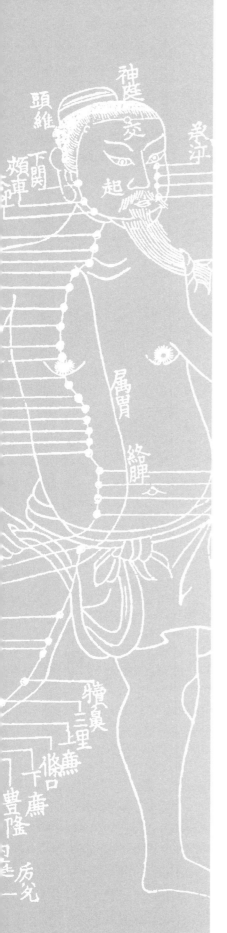

9

KI BREATHING MEDITATION

Ki Breathing meditation is a part of Ki Doin. However, the importance of its practice goes well beyond shiatsu training. I have therefore included it in the final chapter, which focuses on how we can all take responsibility for the health and healing of ourselves and others on a much wider scale.

RESPONDING TO THE EXCESSIVE INTERNALIZATION OF KI

Modern life is full of isolation, insecurity, anxiety, and worry. Developed countries, in particular, exhibit lifestyles that are increasingly self-absorbed and individualistic. When people's lives are lived with such an inward focus, ki becomes increasingly internalized. People from developed nations who visit "developing" countries are often surprised at the lightness and outwardly expressed direction of peoples' ki and way of life. It highlights how excessively internalized the current environment of human relations are.

Having enough money to provide for the necessities of life means that people become increasingly independent units. They no longer need to rely on the help of others. This situation develops the isolation that leads to insecurity. Needing to help and be helped creates a healthy exchange of ki between people. We can live without help from others, but so much is lost—without our even realizing—when this occurs.

HEALING KI RETURNS TO THE GIVER

Practicing the Renki exercises for just fifteen minutes each day will change your ki strength and sensitivity. Heart and body unity deepens, and ki is purified, increasing its healing potential. The Tao heart is the universal heart of nature: it is this heart that creates ki with the greatest healing power for Tao Shiatsu treatment. The Tao heart grows and increases through faith in Tao—Universal Spirit—expressing gratitude for everything that is given and received. Wishing to give one's best for others develops the devotion to express this heart in practical acts. Ultimately the Tao heart brings the realization that nothing is a product of self-ability, that Tao is the force supporting all life. To see this simply as an idealized state, attainable only by the sages or special people, is to miss the opportunity to cultivate and develop your own heart. Of course it requires effort, but it creates the potential for the deepest healing ki to come forth. It is a mistake to think that this is only beneficial for the shiatsu practitioner. Striving to take care of others is the way for all human beings to live the richest lives: the alternative is spending our time calculating how to guarantee only our individual security. What is given unconditionally will return to the giver. This is a universal principle of ki.

KI BREATHING MEDITATION

As a Buddhist practitioner of the Japanese Pure Land sect, for many years my regular practice has been the form of Buddhist chanting called Nembutsu, which invokes the name of Amida Buddha. The purpose of this is to purify the ki of oneself and others. However, it is not necessarily appropriate to recommend this practice to people who have not grown up with this spiritual tradition. As an alternative, then, I would like to recommend Ki Breathing meditation, which can be practiced irrespective of whether you are already following a spiritual practice. It can help anyone to develop greater compassion and bring about healing, because it is based on wishing and hoping for the best for others. This practice came to me one day when I realized that when the focal point of awareness (the ki center) was located at the bottom tanden (two meters below the physical body), the strongest ki was channeled out through the hands. Usually we find in meditation practices that concentration is directed to locations in the physical body such as the abdomen or the nostrils. It was from this observation that the Ki Breathing Method was born.

Practicing ki breathing meditation

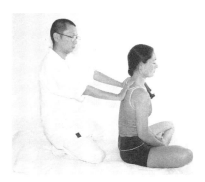

Please try this experiment. Have someone you know (preferably someone you think will enjoy a new and interesting experience) sit down with their back to you. Place your hand on their back.

- Try to empty your mind and not think about anything.
- Drop your point of awareness down to the bottom tanden—just imagine a point approximately two meters below you—and breathe from there.
- The receiver will feel a strong sensation of ki being channeled as you breathe out.

KI BREATHING WITH FIVE STEPS

Include the following principles and try practicing for three minutes. Ask the receiver how it felt.

1. Drop your ki center down to the bottom tanden.
2. Breathe slowly in and out from the bottom tanden.
3. Breathe in and out while visualizing a spiritual symbol—an image, picture, or sign—that most deeply connects you to the universal spirit. Visualize the spiritual symbol expanding to fill the whole of the physical and ki bodies.
4. Pray for the health, happiness, and spiritual growth of others by expanding the symbol so that the whole world and all people are included. Keep trying to infinitely expand the spiritual symbol so that the whole universe and all beings are included.
5. To keep expanding and strengthening the image of the spiritual symbol, and thus deepen the power of the prayer, you must see your heart through the state of naikan, or moment-to-moment awareness.

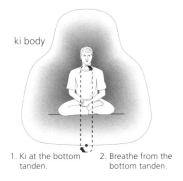

ki body

1. Ki at the bottom tanden.
2. Breathe from the bottom tanden.

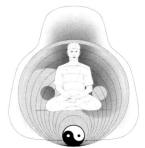

3. Imagine the spiritual symbol at the bottom tanden and expand the image as you breathe.

The meaning of the spiritual symbol, prayer, and naikan

Healing ki comes from the source of all existence. It is never personal. This is the reason for deeply imagining the spiritual symbol: through it we connect to the source of the universe, what the ancient Greeks called To-hen, or the One. The true essence of the universe is not to be found in Quantum Theory, but in the Heart of the Absolute. Lao Tsu, Buddha, Moses, Jesus, Mohammed—all the spiritual masters, saints, and sages—were deeply unified with the source of universal existence. By imagining their image or the symbol associated with the traditions they founded (such as the cross, the lotus flower, or the yin–yang symbol), ki is received from the universal source. From the beginning of Mahayana Buddhism, its practice has been based on the visualization of the Buddha image. However, some of the mystic Buddhist sects also use written characters. Japanese esoteric Buddhist sects imagine the first letter of the Sanskrit alphabet, for example. Therefore the Chinese character Tao, the Hebrew character for God, the Sanskrit letter Om, or whichever traditional symbol is most appropriate and connects you most deeply to the Universal Spirit, should be imagined.

The prayer for "the health and happiness of all beings" is essential. If the exhalation in the breathing method is done with this heart, positive ki is sent to others. When somebody is sick, even if they are separated from you by distance, positive healing ki can be sent to them through this practice. This is the prayer. If the person who is unwell is present, offer this prayer directly. Place your hands at the place where pain is felt and perform Ki Breathing. Saint Paul said in the Bible:

Taoism

Hinduism

Judaism

Buddhism

Christianity

Islam

Animism   Shinto

Symbols of traditional spiritual traditions.

> "And although I have the prophetic gift and see through every secret and through all that may be known, and have sufficient faith to move mountains, but I have no love, I am nothing."
>
> (1 Corinthians 13: 2)

This applies to any spiritual practice. It will remain empty if it lacks the heart of giving the best to others. The existence of each one of us simultaneously contains the wholeness of the universe at every moment. You can also apply this method to yourself if you have any symptom of pain or injury: place your hand on the area to be treated and perform Ki Breathing. Healing ki extends to others and in turn comes back to you. The lesson for everyone is that being stingy or mean-spirited with our physical and mental actions is really the greatest source of unhappiness in our lives.

Naikan, or moment-to-moment awareness, is required as the final principle. This is always necessary for prayer and meditation. The practice of Mahayana Buddhism (and Tao Shiatsu) could be simply said to be "the action of image and naikan." Focusing on your heart, and seeing clearly the image and prayer being expressed, makes it possible to keep increasing the strength of the image of the spiritual symbol and deepening the power of the prayer.

GLOBAL KI UNIFICATION NETWORK

The International Tao Shiatsu Society has created a Global Ki Unification Network. Its aim is to surround the earth with the healing ki of the Uni-

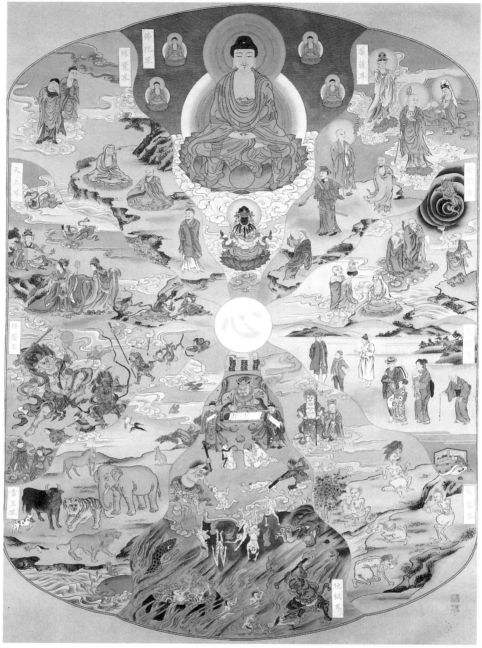

Mandala of Pure Land Buddhism, by Priest Bennei Yamazaki.

versal Spirit. This network hopes to bring the best ki into the lives of all beings, through the practice of Ki Breathing. Members around the world try to devote at least three minutes a day for this purpose. Imagine for a moment how much nicer the world would be if more and more people took responsibility for helping to bring happiness into the lives of others. How much more valuable your life would become by contributing to this!

EPILOGUE

I would like to end this book with the words of Tzvika Calisar, a senior Tao Shiatsu teacher from Israel. He is a humorous person in daily life despite having direct experience of the pain and suffering created by the ongoing conflict of war in the Middle East.

> "Tao Shiatsu can only be practiced by hoping for the best for others. By spreading this wish, people's hearts will shift in a positive way. And they have to shift. I will do anything possible to share Tao Shiatsu, as it is my only hope for the world."

Live with love and humor in your heart. Let Tao Shiatsu grow in our world!

Ryokyu Endo

(英文版) 超指圧
The New Shiatsu Method
―――――――――――――――――――――――――――――――――――――――

2004年4月23日　第1刷発行

著　者	遠藤喨及 マイケル・クリスティーニ、カリサール・ツビカ	印刷・製本所	大日本印刷株式会社
発行者	畑野文夫		
発行所	講談社インターナショナル株式会社 〒112-8652　東京都文京区音羽 1-17-14 電話　03-3944-6493（編集部） 　　　03-3944-6492（営業部・業務部） ホームページ　www.kodansha-intl.co.jp		

落丁本、乱丁本は購入書店名を明記のうえ、講談社インターナショナル業務部宛にお送りください。送料小社負担にてお取替えいたします。なお、この本についてのお問い合わせは、編集部宛にお願いいたします。本書の無断複写（コピー）は著作権法上での例外を除き、禁じられています。

定価はカバーに表示してあります。

© Tao Sangha 2004
Printed in Japan
ISBN4-7700-2990-X